VETERANS: BENEFITS, ISSUES, POLICIES AND PROGRAMS

VETERAN SUICIDE

DATA, ANALYSIS, AND VHA SUICIDE PREVENTION EFFORTS

Veterans: Benefits, Issues, Policies and Programs

Additional books in this series can be found on Nova's website under the Series tab.

Additional E-books in this series can be found on Nova's website under the E-book tab.

Military and Veteran Issues

Additional books in this series can be found on Nova's website under the Series tab.

Additional E-books in this series can be found on Nova's website under the E-book tab.

VETERANS: BENEFITS, ISSUES, POLICIES AND PROGRAMS

VETERAN SUICIDE

DATA, ANALYSIS, AND VHA SUICIDE PREVENTION EFFORTS

ISMAEL O. WALKER
AND
JILLIAN C. GRAY
EDITORS

New York

For permission to use material from this book please contact us:
Telephone 631-231-7269; Fax 631-231-8175
Web Site: http://www.novapublishers.com

LIBRARY OF CONGRESS CATALOGING-IN-PUBLICATION DATA

ISBN: 978-1-62618-548-7

Published by Nova Science Publishers, Inc. † New York

CONTENTS

PREFACE

The 2012 Suicide Data Report contains prevalence data and characteristics of suicide among Veterans and evidence of change in outcomes among Veterans at risk for suicide. This book provides an overview and analysis of information collected through collaborative data sharing agreements with U.S. states, reports of non-fatal suicide events among Veterans using VHA services and analysis of data obtained from the Veterans Crisis Line.

Chapter 1 – The 2012 Suicide Data Report contains prevalence data and characteristics of suicide among Veterans and evidence of change in outcomes among Veterans at risk for suicide. Included in this report are an overview and analysis of information collected through collaborative data sharing agreements with U.S. states, reports of non-fatal suicide events among Veterans using VHA services and analysis of data obtained from the Veterans Crisis Line.

VHA acknowledges the strengths and limitations of the report, which provided early findings of the suicide data project and related data and agrees with the conclusions of the report.

Chapter 2 – In 2007, the Department of Veterans Affairs began an intensive effort to reduce suicide among Veterans. This effort had its roots in the Mental Health staffing expansion and the Joshua Omvig Bill, and it included both attention to Veterans in crisis as well as those determined to be at high risk for suicide. The effort also included the development of data systems to increase understanding of suicide among Veterans and inform both the VA and other suicide prevention programs. Information on the characteristics and outcomes of Veterans at risk for suicide is critical to the development of improved suicide prevention programs.

In 2008, VA's Mental Health Services established a suicide surveillance and clinical support system based on reports of suicide and suicide events (i.e. non-fatal attempts, serious suicide ideation, suicide plan) submitted by Suicide Prevention Coordinators located at each VA Medical Center and large outpatient facility. In addition to information obtained from suicide behavior reports, data on the characteristics and outcomes of callers to the national toll-free Veterans Crisis Line – a universally available crisis intervention resource – are available. In 2010, the VA also began an intensive effort to shorten delays associated with access to NDI data and increase understanding of suicide among all Veterans by developing data sharing agreements with all 50 U.S. states. The integration of information collected through the NDI, state mortality records, Suicide Behavior Reports, Veterans Crisis Line, and the VA's universal electronic medical records contribute to an increased understanding of suicide and risk management by identifying gaps in existing knowledge, opportunities for intervention and the impact of VA-sponsored suicide prevention programs.

All of these data collection systems have matured to the point where they can now begin to provide VA with information that can be used to both determine if the current suicide prevention program is having an effect, where gaps may occur, and provide direction for the future. This report is an initial attempt to look at all of this information together in order to provide an overall picture of Veteran suicide to drive suicide prevention program development and improve outcomes for Veterans at risk for suicide. It is expected that reporting will be refined as time goes on and more data become available. This report contains a systematic overview of data obtained from the State Mortality Project, Suicide Behavior Reports for fiscal years 2009 – 2012, and Veterans Crisis Line.

Chapter 3 - Responsibility for prevention of veteran suicide lies primarily with the Veterans Health Administration (VHA), within the Department of Veterans Affairs (VA). The VHA Strategic Plan for Suicide Prevention is based on a public health framework, which has three major components: (1) surveillance, (2) risk and protective factors, and (3) prevention interventions.

No nationwide surveillance system exists for suicide among all veterans; therefore, the actual incidence of suicide among veterans is not known. Surveillance, or systematic collection of data on completed (i.e., fatal) suicides, is essential to define the scope of the problem (i.e., the suicide rate among veterans), identify characteristics associated with higher or lower risk of suicide, and track changes in the suicide rate over time to evaluate suicide prevention interventions. In the absence of a nationwide surveillance system for veteran suicide, the VHA is attempting to determine the rate of suicide among veterans in two ways, both in collaboration with the Centers for Disease Control and Prevention (CDC).

Information collected in surveillance is used to identify suicide risk factors (i.e., characteristics associated with higher rates of suicide) and protective factors (i.e., characteristics associated with lower rates of suicide). This is essential in order to design interventions that reduce risk factors and/or increase protective factors, thus lowering overall risk of suicide. Risk factors are also helpful in identifying at-risk groups or individuals so that interventions can be delivered to the people who need them most. Within the VHA, this research is supported by the Office of Research and Development; a Center of Excellence in suicide prevention; and a Mental Illness Research, Education, and Clinical Center on suicide prevention.

The intervention cycle includes three stages: design and test interventions, implement interventions, and evaluate interventions. The research components mentioned above have roles in small-scale pilot testing and large-scale evaluations of interventions. This report discusses seven areas of VHA suicide prevention interventions: (1) easy access to care, (2) education, (3) screening and treatment, (4) limited access to lethal means, (5) suicide hotline, (6) media restrictions, and (7) suicide prevention coordinators.

This report identifies challenges the VHA faces in each component of suicide prevention and discusses potential issues for Congress. A recurring theme is the need for the VHA to work in concert with other federal, state, and local government agencies; private for-profit and not-forprofit health care providers; veterans, their families, and their communities; and other individuals or organizations that might be able to help. Specific challenges in surveillance include timeliness of data, accurate identification of decedents as veterans, and consistent classification of deaths as suicides. Challenges in risk and protective factors research include a need for more collaboration and dialogue among agencies involved in suicide prevention and across other areas of public health (because suicide has some of the same risk and protective factors as other public health problems). Challenges in VHA suicide prevention interventions also include the need for more collaboration and dialogue, as well as an apparent gap between policy and practice, and misperceptions about mental illness and mental health care.

In: Veteran Suicide
Editors: I. O. Walker and J. C. Gray
ISBN: 978-1-62618-548-7

Chapter 1

2012 Suicide Data Report: Veterans Health Administration Response and Executive Summary*

Robert A. Petzel

The 2012 Suicide Data Report contains prevalence data and characteristics of suicide among Veterans and evidence of change in outcomes among Veterans at risk for suicide. Included in this report are an overview and analysis of information collected through collaborative data sharing agreements with U.S. states, reports of non-fatal suicide events among Veterans using VHA services and analysis of data obtained from the Veterans Crisis Line.

VHA acknowledges the strengths and limitations of the report, which provided early findings of the suicide data project and related data and agrees with the conclusions of the report.

Data collected through the Department of Veterans Affairs' (VA) initiatives identify opportunities for the continued support and development of new prevention programs. Major findings of the report include:

- While the percentage of all suicides reported as Veterans has decreased, the number of suicides has increased.

---

* This report was released by the Department of Veterans Affairs, February 2013.

- A majority of Veteran suicides are among those age 50 years and older. Male Veterans who die by suicide are older than non-Veteran males who die by suicide.
- The age distribution of Veteran and non-Veterans women who have died from suicide is similar.
- The demographic characteristics of Veterans who have died from suicide are similar among those with and without a history of VHA service use.
- Among those at risk, the first 4 weeks following service require intensive monitoring and case management (which verifies the importance of the Enhanced Care Package for those at high risk).
- There is preliminary evidence in 2012 indicating a decrease in the rate of nonfatal suicide events for VHA utilizing Veterans.
- Decreasing rates of non-fatal suicide events are associated with increasing age.
- The data show a decrease in the 12 month re-event prevalence in fiscal year (FY) 2012.
- The majority of Veterans who have a suicide event were last seen in an outpatient setting. A high prevalence of non-fatal suicide events result from overdose or other intentional poisoning.
- Continued increases in calls to the Veterans Crisis Line may be associated with efforts to enhance awareness of VHA services through public education campaigns.
- The majority of callers to the Veterans Crisis Line are male and between the ages of 50-59.
- Differences in the age composition of callers to the Veterans Crisis Line are associated with gender.
- A large percentage of callers to the Veterans Crisis Line are identified as Veterans.
- Approximately 19 percent of callers to the Veterans Crisis Line call more than once each month.
- The percentage of callers to the Veterans Crisis Line who are currently thinking of suicide has decreased.
- The percentage of all calls resulting in a rescue has decreased, indicating that the calls are less emergent and callers are using the Crisis Line earlier.
- The percentage of callers receiving a referral for follow-up care is increasing

- Approximately 93 percent of all Veterans Crisis Line referrals are made to callers with a history of VHA service use in the past 12 months.
- Service use continues to increase following a referral for care.
- Between FY 2009 — FY 2011, use of inpatient and outpatient services increased following a rescue.
- The 12 month re-event prevalence has decreased among those who have been rescued or received a referral for follow-up care.

Although this was not a research-based analysis and there are significant limitations in the data that are available, as described in the report, this first attempt at a comprehensive review of Veteran suicide does provide us with valuable information for future directions in care and program development. While the numbers of Veterans who die from suicide each day has remained relatively stable over the past 12 years (varying from 18 -22 per day), the percentage of people who die by suicide in America who are Veterans has decreased slightly. At the same time, the number of Americans who die by suicide each day has increased. This provides preliminary evidence that the programs initiated by VA are improving outcomes. VA must continue to provide a high level of care, and recognize that there is still much more work to do. As long as Veterans die by suicide, we must continue to improve and provide even better services and care. This report provides us with valuable information about opportunities to do even better work and take further action.

VA has indentified the following immediate actions to take in response to the report: *Action #1:* A taskforce designed to provide recommendations for innovating mental health care in VA has been established and will be given this report to help guide its work. A report from this inter-agency group will be forthcoming to the inter-agency task force developed to implement President Obama's Mental Health Executive Order, which is highly focused on suicide prevention. The work of this group includes developing action plans to address risk in a broader sense for all patients in both mental health and non-mental health settings. This includes reassessing the value of traditional suicide risk assessments and screening (which is done now extensively in VA), and adding ways to identify life stressors and concerns earlier. Improving risk identification through these alternative approaches and increasing the numbers of Veterans who are engaged in the enhanced follow-up program may address that identified sensitive time period following VA contact as an outpatient as well as for inpatients. A full report with risk identification strategies and patient-centered focused care options will be provided no later than March 1, 2013, to VA's Under Secretary for Health.

Action #2: Population groups indentified in the report that require additional interventions and engagement include women Veterans and Vietnam Era Veterans. Additional VA training programs will be developed targeting providers of these groups of patients and Suicide Prevention Coordinators will be provided materials to do "refresher" training on suicide risk awareness and risk assessment for all staff. These materials will be developed and released to the field no later than June 1, 2013.

Action #3: Outreach remains critically important. Knowing that VA treatment strategies are effective provides an impetus to get more Veterans involved in treatment programs earlier. Maintaining the availability of the Veterans Crisis Line to address all areas of concern for Veterans is valuable, Our communication and outreach strategies appear to be effective in this area -- we should continue our work and expand in this area. This is an on-going action item and congruent with the milestones currently set in the Mental Health Executive Order.

Action #4: VA recognizes its role and responsibility in maintaining the safety and wellbeing of our Nation's Veterans of all eras. We will diligently continue to pursue successful and effective interventions for those Veterans at risk for suicide and those suffering from mental health related concerns through research and practice, using all available information and data. We will continue to add to this information base as data continues to become available and provide updates to this on-going report. This is an on-going action item. A follow-up to this report is expected in May of 2013 as the VA/Department of Defense Suicide Repository is completed and additional data from the Centers for Disease Control and Prevention is obtained and analyzed.

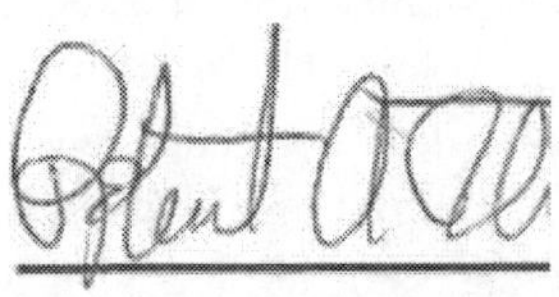

Robert A. Petzel, M.D.
Under Secretary for Health

In: Veteran Suicide
Editors: I. O. Walker and J. C. Gray
ISBN: 978-1-62618-548-7

Chapter 2

SUICIDE DATA REPORT, 2012*

Janet Kemp and Robert Bossarte

LIST OF ABBREVIATIONS

VA	Department of Veterans Affairs
NDI	National Death Index
VHA	Veterans Health Administration
DoD	Department of Defense
VCL	Veterans Crisis Line
SPAN	Suicide Prevention and Application Network
DoDSER	Department of Defense's Suicide Event Reporting system

INTRODUCTION

In 2007, the Department of Veterans Affairs began an intensive effort to reduce suicide among Veterans. This effort had its roots in the Mental Health staffing expansion and the Joshua Omvig Bill, and it included both attention to Veterans in crisis as well as those determined to be at high risk for suicide. The effort also included the development of data systems to increase understanding of suicide among Veterans and inform both the VA and other suicide prevention programs. Information on the characteristics and outcomes

* This report was released by the Department of Veterans Affairs, February 2013.

of Veterans at risk for suicide is critical to the development of improved suicide prevention programs.

In 2008, VA's Mental Health Services established a suicide surveillance and clinical support system based on reports of suicide and suicide events (i.e. non-fatal attempts, serious suicide ideation, suicide plan) submitted by Suicide Prevention Coordinators located at each VA Medical Center and large outpatient facility. In addition to information obtained from suicide behavior reports, data on the characteristics and outcomes of callers to the national toll-free Veterans Crisis Line – a universally available crisis intervention resource – are available. In 2010, the VA also began an intensive effort to shorten delays associated with access to NDI data and increase understanding of suicide among all Veterans by developing data sharing agreements with all 50 U.S. states. The integration of information collected through the NDI, state mortality records, Suicide Behavior Reports, Veterans Crisis Line, and the VA's universal electronic medical records contribute to an increased understanding of suicide and risk management by identifying gaps in existing knowledge, opportunities for intervention and the impact of VA-sponsored suicide prevention programs.

All of these data collection systems have matured to the point where they can now begin to provide VA with information that can be used to both determine if the current suicide prevention program is having an effect, where gaps may occur, and provide direction for the future. This report is an initial attempt to look at all of this information together in order to provide an overall picture of Veteran suicide to drive suicide prevention program development and improve outcomes for Veterans at risk for suicide. It is expected that reporting will be refined as time goes on and more data become available. This report contains a systematic overview of data obtained from the State Mortality Project, Suicide Behavior Reports for fiscal years 2009 – 2012, and Veterans Crisis Line.

State Mortality Data Project

Up to this point the primary source for Veteran suicide information has been limited to those Veterans who receive care in VA. Information on the rate and characteristics of suicide among those who used VHA services is available for the fiscal years 2001—2009 based on information from analyses of mortality data obtained through the National Death Index. Using this information we have identified a decrease in the age-adjusted rate of suicide (per 100,000 person years) between the fiscal years 2001--2003 and relative stability in suicide rates during recent years (Figure 1).

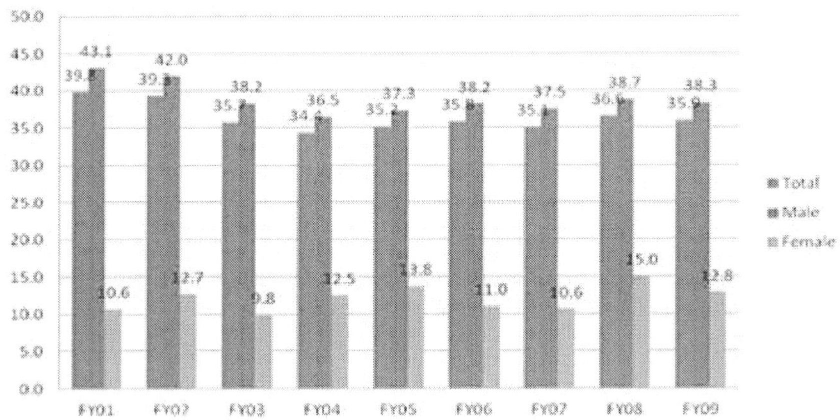

Figure 1. Suicide Rates Among VHA Users by Sex and Fiscal Year.

While data obtained from NDI provide a reliable mechanism for identifying suicides among some Veterans, these data often encounter lengthy delays and require a population list to identify cause of death information. The Department of Veterans Affairs believes that a comprehensive suicide prevention program requires timely and accurate information beyond that acquired from its internal patient population.

It was determined that additional data on Veterans with and without history of VHA service use, among those who have accessed crisis services, and for those with report of non-fatal suicide events are needed to overcome delays associated in acquisition of mortality data, improve understanding of suicide among all Veterans, and identify changes in outcomes among those who use receive care from the VHA. The need for comprehensive information led to the decision to seek support from state governments for a collaborative effort to improve current understanding of suicide among Veterans among Veterans with and without history of VHA service use. In 2010, Secretary Shinseki engaged Governors of all U.S. states requesting support and collaboration to improve the timeliness and utility of suicide mortality reporting. The Secretary's request asked each state to designate a point of contact who would work with the VISN 2 Center of Excellence for Suicide Prevention to develop data use agreements for the purpose of sharing identified mortality data for all known suicides. The time frame for the original request for data included all known suicides reported between January 1, 1999 and December 31, 2004.

However, following discussion of developing program needs, the time frame was extended for each data request including existing and pending data use agreements that share individually identifiable data through December 31, 2015.

Data obtained from states is currently being used to assess the reliability and validity of Veteran information collected during mortality reporting, fulfill requirements of PL111.163 to determine the number of Veterans who have died from suicide (1999-2009), and to identify opportunities to improve the timeliness and utility of suicide reporting. Currently, all 50 U.S. states include some information on the decedent's history of U.S. military service. A complete listing of Veteran identifiers by state and project year has been provided as Appendix A.

Project Cost

The cumulative cost of the State Mortality Data Project has been $46,771.29 as of 11/16/2012; including FY12 expenditures of $35,094.23 and FY13 expenditures of $11,677.06. All costs associated with the State Mortality Data Project are related to state fees for processing and delivery of mortality data.

Project Status

As of November 2012, data have been received from 34 states and data use agreements have been approved by an additional eight states. Data will be received from these states once the terms of individual data use and financial arrangements are finalized. An additional 11 states and territories have not made a decision regarding our request or are in the process of developing Data Use Agreements for VA review.

A total of five states and territories have requested modifications to the initial request for data sharing or have been unable to identify an internal point of contact to support this program. Efforts to address initial concerns and/or identify appropriate contacts within non-participating areas are ongoing. While the State Mortality Project has not finalized contributions from all states, evaluation of existing data determined that the pilot effort has reached a point of statistical significance allowing for analysis of available data.

Availability of data by state is listed in Table 1 and an estimated schedule for updates to the existing data has been provided as Appendix B.

Recently, efforts to obtain information on deaths from suicide for Veterans have expanded to several U.S. territories including Guam, Puerto Rico, US Virgin Islands, Commonwealth of Northern Mariana Islands, and American Samoa as well as the Philippines, due to the presence of a VA facility and a large population of US Military Veterans in these regions. The Department of State has also been approached about obtaining information on suicide deaths among Americans living in foreign territories. Data availability and the status of each data request are summarized in Table 1.

To date, data from twenty-one (21) states have been cleaned and entered into a single integrated file containing information on more than 147,000 suicides and 27,062 reported Veterans.

In addition to the issues identified above, barriers to full project implementation include inconsistent availability of requested information in all states, barriers to providing non-resident data and sending preference to provide de-identified data due to conflicting interpretations of Social Security laws. Negotiations with states are continuing as we begin requesting more recent years' data as well as renewing or revising previously completed Data Use Agreements.

Table 1. Status of Data Request/Availability by State

State/Area	1999	2000	2001	2002	2003	2004	2005	2006	2007	2008	2009	2010	2011
Alabama	I	I	I	I	I	I	I	I	I	I	I	I	P
Alaska	I	I	I	I	I	I	I	I	I	I	I	I	P
American Samoa	R	R	R	R	R	R	R	R	R	R	R	R	R
Arizona	R	R	R	R	R	R	R	R	R	R	R	R	R
Arkansas	A	A	A	A	A	A	A	A	A	A	A	A	A
California	P	P	P	P	P	P	P	P	P	P	P	P	P
Common wealth N. Mariana Islands	R	R	R	R	R	R	R	R	R	R	R	R	R
Colorado	K	K	K	K	K	K	K	K	K	K	K	K	P
Connecticut	P	P	A	A	A	A	A	A	A	A	A	P	P
Delaware	R	R	R	R	R	R	R	R	R	R	R	R	R
Florida	I	I	I	I	I	I	I	I	I	I	I	I	I

Table 1. (Continued)

State/Area	1999	2000	2001	2002	2003	2004	2005	2006	2007	2008	2009	2010	2011
Georgia	P	P	P	P	P	I	I	I	I	I	I	I	I
Guam	R	R	R	R	R	R	R	R	R	R	R	R	R
Hawaii	A	A	A	A	A	A	A	A	A	A	A	A	P
Idaho	I	I	I	I	I	I	I	I	I	I	I	I	P
Illinois	R	R	R	R	R	R	R	R	R	R	R	R	R
Indiana	C	C	C	C	C	C	C	C	C	C	C	C	C
Iowa	P	P	P	P	P	P	P	P	P	P	P	P	P
Kansas	I	I	I	I	I	I	I	I	I	I	I	I	P
Kentucky	R	R	R	R	R	R	R	R	R	R	R	R	R
Louisiana	A	A	A	A	A	A	A	A	A	A	A	A	P
Maine	I	I	I	I	I	I	I	I	I	I	I	P	P
Maryland	R	R	R	R	R	R	R	R	R	R	R	R	R
Massachusetts	I	I	I	I	I	I	I	I	I	I	P	P	P
Michigan	I	I	I	I	I	I	I	I	I	I	I	I	P
Minnesota	I	I	I	I	I	I	I	I	I	I	I	I	P
Mississippi	P	P	P	P	P	P	P	P	P	P	P	P	P
Missouri	I	I	I	I	I	I	I	I	I	I	I	P	P
Montana	A	A	A	A	A	A	A	A	A	A	A	A	P
Nebraska	I	I	I	I	I	I	I	I	I	I	I	I	P
Nevada	I	I	I	I	I	I	I	I	I	I	I	I	P
New Hampshire	P	P	P	P	P	P	P	P	P	P	P	P	P
New Jersey	I	I	I	I	I	I	I	I	I	I	I	I	P
New Mexico	P	P	P	P	P	P	P	P	P	P	P	P	P
New York	I	I	I	I	I	I	I	I	I	I	I	I	P
New York City	I	I	I	I	I	I	I	I	I	I	I	I	P
North Carolina	I	I	I	I	I	I	I	I	I	I	I	I	I
North Dakota	A	A	A	A	A	A	A	A	A	A	A	A	P
Ohio	K	K	K	K	K	K	K	K	K	K	K	K	K
Oklahoma	I	I	I	I	I	I	I	I	I	I	I	P	P
Oregon	A	A	A	A	A	A	A	A	A	A	A	A	P
Pennsylvania	I	I	I	I	I	I	I	I	I	I	I	I	P
Philippines	R	R	R	R	R	R	R	R	R	R	R	R	R
Puerto Rico	R	R	R	R	R	R	R	R	R	R	R	R	R
Rhode Island	R	R	R	R	R	R	R	R	R	R	R	R	R
South Carolina	C	C	C	C	C	C	C	C	C	C	C	C	C
South Dakota	P	P	P	P	P	P	P	P	P	P	P	P	P
State Department	R	R	R	R	R	R	R	R	R	R	R	R	R

State/Area	1999	2000	2001	2002	2003	2004	2005	2006	2007	2008	2009	2010	2011
Tennessee	R	R	R	R	R	R	R	R	R	R	R	R	R
Texas	K	K	K	K	K	K	K	K	K	K	K	K	P
Utah	A	A	A	A	A	A	A	A	A	A	A	A	A
Vermont	I	I	I	I	I	I	I	I	I	I	I	I	P
Virgin Islands	R	R	R	R	R	R	R	R	R	R	R	R	R
Virginia	K	K	K	K	K	K	K	K	K	K	K	A	A
Washington	I	I	I	I	I	I	I	I	I	I	I	I	I
Washington D.C.	P	P	P	P	P	P	P	P	P	P	P	P	P
West Virginia	I	I	I	I	I	I	I	I	I	I	I	I	P
Wisconsin	A	P	A	A	A	A	A	A	A	A	A	A	P
Wyoming	P	P	P	P	P	P	P	P	P	P	P	P	P

I= data included in report,
A= available for future analysis,
P= pending state approval/processing,
R = requested but not received,
C= being processed,
K = provided partial information

Reliability and Validity of Veteran Identifiers

A previous assessment of Veteran identifiers on Colorado death certificates suggested that the reliability of Veteran identifiers on state death certificates is acceptable.[1] The state mortality project offers a unique opportunity to more directly quantify the misclassification of Veteran status as indicated on death certificates for suicide. A preliminary assessment of data collected from *Washington State (Washington initially provided data from 1999-2008)* as part of this project supports conclusions of acceptable reliability reported in previous assessments and demonstrates the utility of using VA administrative data for confirming service history.

Comparing the death certificate indicator in Washington to VA and DOD records, 5% misclassification was observed overall, suggesting that death certificate reporting is a reasonable indicator of Veteran status among suicide deaths that could be used to track the overall rate of Veteran suicides. However, misclassification was considerably higher among validated Veterans with 11% of true Veterans classified as non-Veterans on the death certificate. Only 2% of true non-Veterans were misclassified as Veterans on the death certificate. The ability of death certificates to fully capture female Veterans was particularly low; only 67% of true female Veterans were identified. Younger or unmarried

Veterans and those with lower levels of education were also more likely to be missed on the death certificate. This decreased sensitivity in specific subgroups can affect both suicide surveillance and research efforts that utilize Veteran status on the death certificate. From a surveillance standpoint, the rate of Veteran suicides will be underestimated in these groups. From a research standpoint, the generalizability of study findings for specific subgroups may be limited. This preliminary analysis demonstrates the value of linking information from state mortality record obtained through data sharing agreements and VA and DoD administrative files.

Main Finding: Continued research on the reliability and validity of Veteran identifiers is needed.

Limitations of Existing Data

Currently available data include information on suicide mortality among the population of residents in 21 states. Veteran status in each of these areas is determined by a single question asking about history of U.S. military service. Information about history of military service is routinely obtained from family members and collected by funeral home staff and has not been validated using information from the DoD or VA. Further, Veteran status was not collected by each state during each year of the project period. Appendix B provides a listing of the availability of Veteran identifiers by state and year.

Further, this report contains information from the first 21 states to contribute data for this project and does not include some states, such as California and Texas, with larger Veteran populations. Information from these states has been received and will be included in future reports.

Suicide among Veterans – As Reported on Death Certificates

Of the 147,763 suicides reported in 21 states, 27,062 (18.3%) were identified as having history of U.S. military service on death certificates. However, Veteran status was unknown or not reported for more than 23% (n=34,027) of all suicides during the project period. Without linking to VA or DoD resources to validate history of U.S. military service, it is necessary to remove those without information on history of military service from estimates of Veteran status among suicide decedents. Among cases where history of U.S. military service was reported, Veterans comprised approximately 22.2%

of all suicides reported during the project period. If this prevalence estimate is assumed to be constant across all U.S. states, an estimated 22 Veterans will have died from suicide each day in the calendar year 2010. As Veteran status on death certificates is verified in on-going work the overall percentage remains comparable. As shown in Appendix C, preliminary data for the 2012 calendar year will be available from a limited number of participating states within the next 12 months. It is important to note that estimates of the number of Veterans who died from suicide are based on information reported on state death certificates and may be subject to reporting error. It is recommended that the estimated number of Veterans be interpreted with caution due to the use of data from a sample of states and existing evidence of uncertainty in Veteran identifiers on U.S. death certificates. *It is important to note that both Veteran populations and those who die by suicide are significantly more likely to be male.* According to data provided by the United States Census Bureau, 93% of all Veterans are male and 21% of all males aged 18 years and older have history of U.S. military service. Further, history of U.S. military service increases with age, with the highest percentage of Veterans aged 55 years and older.[2] Information reported on state death certificates indicates that the ages 50-59 years is also an important group for addressing risk for suicide. Between 1999 and 2010 the average age of male Veterans who died from suicide was 59.6 years among Veterans identified on state death certificates and 54.5 years among those who could be validated using VA administrative records. The average age of male Veterans who died from suicide was considerably older than the average age of male suicide decedents who were not identified as Veterans (43.1 years). For example, according to data provided by the Centers for Disease Control and Prevention (2010), approximately 79% of all suicides among adults aged 18 years and older were male and approximately 44% of all male suicides were among those aged 50 years of age and older. [3] It is therefore possible that epidemiologic characteristic of suicide in the general population (i.e. higher rates of suicide among older adult males) may contribute to a comparatively high prevalence of Veterans among those who die from suicide.

Main Finding: While the percentage of all suicides reported as Veteran has decreased, the number of suicides has increased.

As shown in Figure 2, the percentage of all suicides identified as Veteran declined between the years 1999-2003 and has remained comparatively constant over recent years. However, the number of deaths by suicide has increased. Between 2007 and 2010, the number of deaths from suicide in the U.S. increased by nearly 11% and the rate of suicide increased by over 8%.

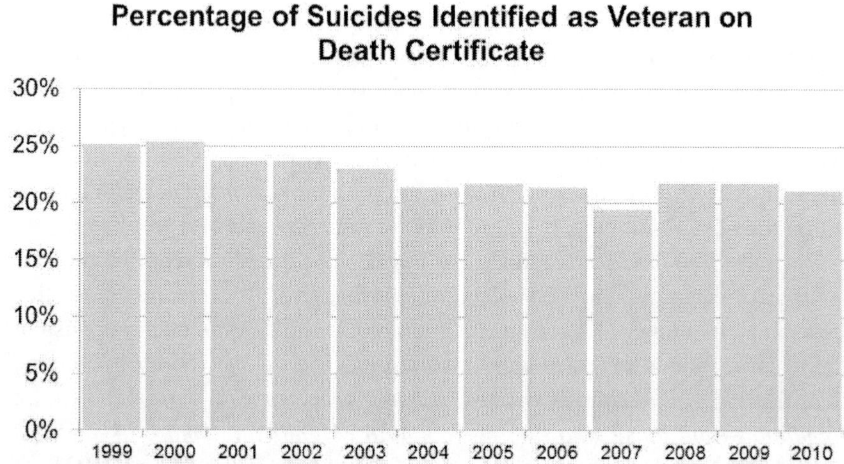

Veteran Status Missing from Death Certificate – Maine, North Carolina, Massachusetts, West Virginia, Oklahoma (1999-2003), Nebraska (1999-2004), Minnesota (2010)

Figure 2. Percentage of Suicides Identified as Veteran by Year 1999-2010.

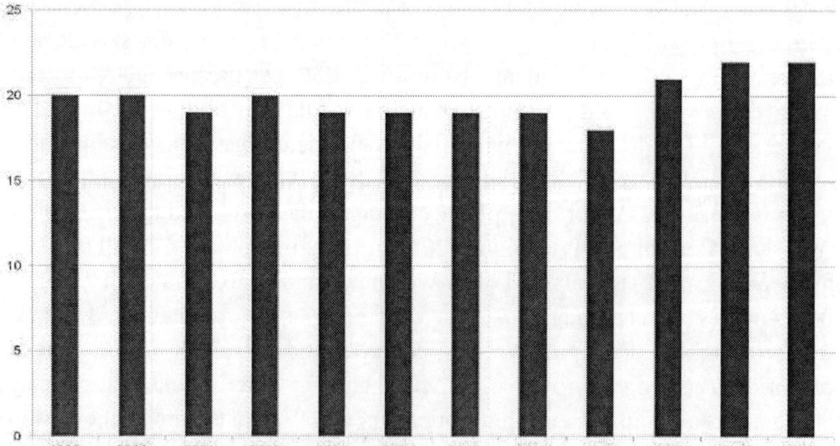

Figure 3. Estimated Number of Veteran Suicides per day by Year.

Estimates that the number of suicides among Veterans each day has increased, are based on information provided by 21 states and may not be generalizable to the larger Veteran population. To account for uncertainty in the estimated number of Veterans who have died from suicide each year, confidence intervals were calculated using variability in the percentage of

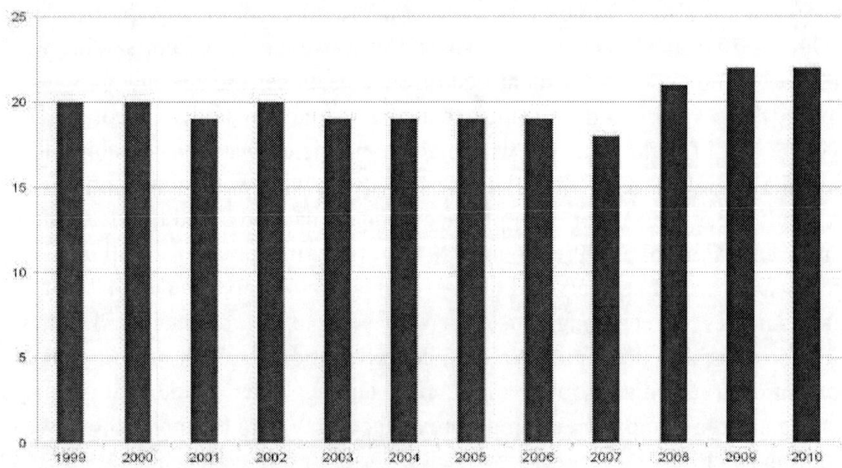

Veterans reported among all suicides in participating states. Information on the estimated count and lower and upper limits for the estimate for each year has been provided in Table 2.

Table 2. Estimated Number of Veteran Suicides and Confidence Intervals by Year

Year 1999	Estimated Count 20	Lower Limit 19	Upper Limit 20
2000	20	19	20
2001	19	19	19
2002	20	19	20
2003	19	19	19
2004	19	18	19
2005	19	18	19
2006	19	18	19
2007	18	17	18
2008	21	20	21
2009	22	21	22
2010	22	21	22

The estimated number of Veterans who died from suicide each day was calculated as the percentage of all suicides identified as Veterans multiplied by the number of suicides in the U.S. and divided by the number of days in a year. The estimated number of Veterans who have died from suicide is based on data obtained from 21 states and has been calculated using service history as reported on death certificates. An assessment of Veteran status on Washington State death certificates identified a measureable amount of error among those with history of U.S. military service. Therefore, estimates of the number of Veterans who have died from suicide each day based on proxy report of history of U.S. military service should be interpreted with caution..

It is also possible to estimate the excess burden of suicide among Veterans by comparing the percentages of Veterans in the general population and the percentage of Veterans among those who have died from suicide. Figures 4 & 5 show the percentage of Veterans living in the first 21 states to contribute to this project and the estimated prevalence of Veterans among suicide decedents in those same areas for males and females respectively. As shown in Figures 4 & 5, difference in the population percentage of male Veterans in 21 participating states and the percentage of Veterans among males who died from suicide in those same areas is highest among younger Veterans and decreases with age. However, the difference between the population percentage of female Veterans and female Veterans who died from suicide in those same areas is greater than it is for males and does not decrease with age. (Please note that these two Figures use different scales. The two populations are very different in regards to numbers and different scales are needed to demonstrate the differences in each.)

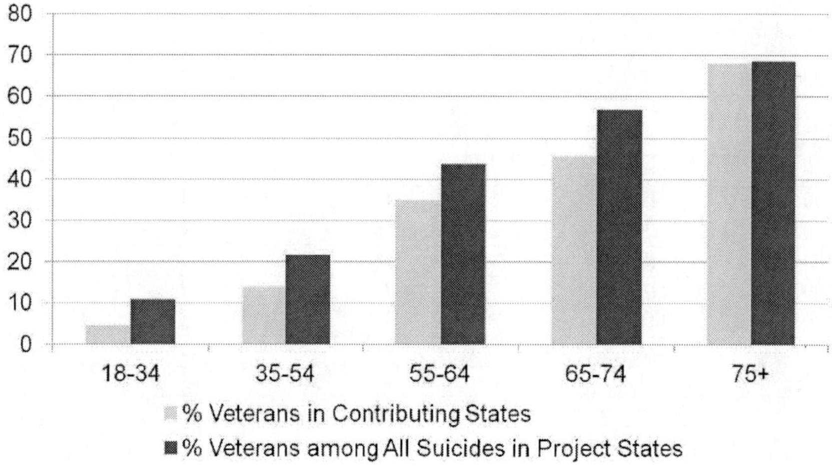

Figure 4. Percentage of Male Veterans in 21 States and among Those Who Died from Suicide.

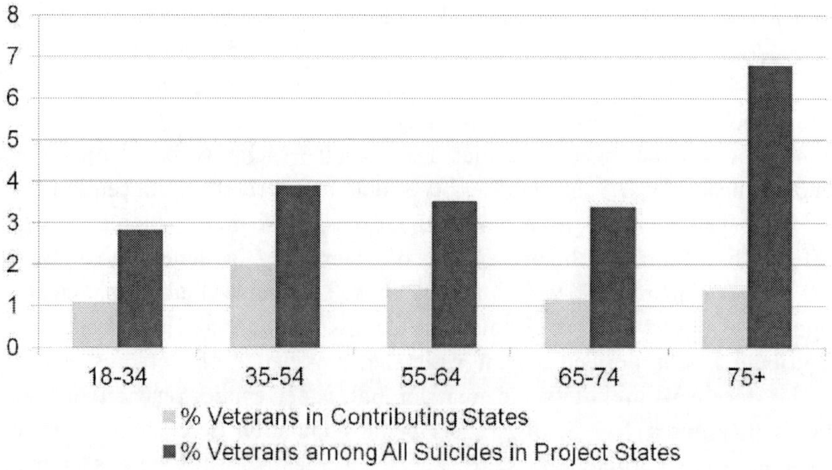

Figure 5. Percentage of Female Veterans in 21 States and among Those Who Died from Suicide.

An important assumption underlying current estimates of the number of Veteran suicides in the total population is stability in the percentage of Veterans among suicides reported in each state. As shown Figure 6, there is variability in this percentage of Veterans among all suicides across states during the project period; with the percentage of Veteran suicides ranging from a low of just over 7% to more than 26% of all suicides. Available data prevent any firm conclusions about correlates or causes of difference in the prevalence of Veteran suicides in each area. However, the observed variability in the percentage of all suicides reported as Veteran across states suggests that this number is not constant across areas. It is possible that differences in demographic composition and service availability contribute to variability in Veteran suicide across geographic regions. Additional study of the causes and correlates of variability in Veteran suicide across communities is recommended.

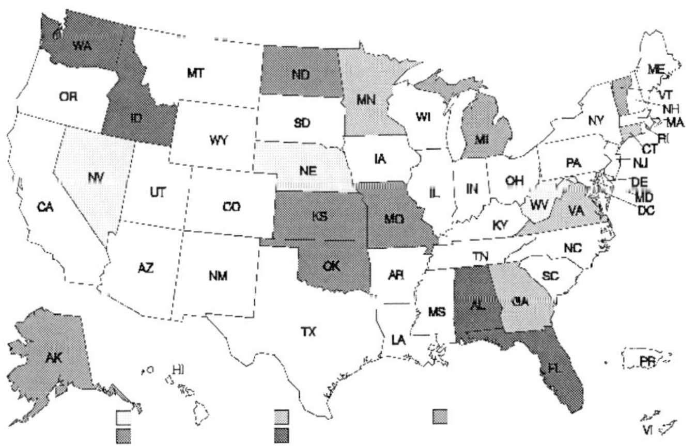

*Among states reporting Veteran status.

Figure 6. Percentage of Suicides Identified as Veteran by State.*

Veteran Status and Demographic Characteristics among Suicide Decedents

Table 3 shows the percentage of suicides across 10-year age groups for all Veterans, Veterans with history of VHA service use, and those without report of military service (non-Veterans). As shown in Table 3, those identified as

Veterans of U.S. military service were more likely to be aged 50 years and older than those without report of military service. Specifically, more than 69% of all Veteran suicides were among those aged 50 years and older, compared to approximately 37% among those who were not identified as Veterans. The final two columns in Table 3 list the Chi-Square values and p-statistics comparing the age distributions of non-Veterans, Veterans, and Veterans with history of VHA service use in the year before their death. These comparisons suggest that those identified as Veterans were significantly more likely to be age 50 years and older when compared to those without indication of military service. Further, those with history of VHA service use were more likely than other Veterans to be between the ages of 50 – 79 years.

Table 3. Percentage of Suicides by Age and Veteran Status

Age Group	Non-Veteran	Veteran	VHA Veteran	, p (1)	, p (2)
29 years and younger	21.6%	6.0%	3.0%	3902.36, <.0001	83.38, <.0001
30 – 39 years	19.3%	9.1%	5.2%	1386.39, <.0001	110.38, <.0001
40 – 49 years	24.5%	15.6%	14.0%	833.21, <.0001	12.34, 0.01
50 – 59 years	18.2%	20.0%	23.4%	63.54, <.0001	48.00, <.0001
60 – 69 years	8.1%	16.5%	19.6%	1655.55, <.0001	43.23, <.0001
70 – 79 years	4.6%	18.6%	20.0%	5592.63, <.0001	6.64, 0.01
80 years and older	3.7%	14.2%	14.8%	3980.27, <.0001	0.21, 0.65

(1) Veteran (as indicated on death certificate) compared to non-Veteran.

(2) Veteran with VHA service use compared to general population of Veterans. (as indicated on death certificate)

Main Finding: More than 69% of Veteran suicides are among those age 50 years and older.

There is evidence of differences in gender composition among Veterans who have died from suicide when compared to those without history of military service. Specifically, males accounted for more than 97% of all suicides among those identified as Veterans, compared to approximately 74% among non-Veteran suicide decedents (Table 4). Differences in the distribution of age between males with and without report of military service are consistent with trends identified in the larger population of suicide decedents. As shown in Table 5, females accounted for less than 3% of all suicides among reported Veterans, compared to more than 26% among suicide decedents without a reported history of military service. Overall, there were few differences in the age distribution of suicide decedents with and without report of military service.

Table 4. Percentage of Suicides by Age and Veteran Status among Males

Age Group	Non-Veteran	Veteran	VHA Veteran	, p (1)	, p (2)
29 years and younger	24.4%	5.8%	2.9%	4654.56,	79.60,
				<.0001	<.0001
30 – 39 years	20.0%	8.9%	4.9%	1525.62,	109.07,
				<.0001	<.0001
40 – 49 years	23.5%	15.0%	13.2%	709.62,	15.59,
				<.0001	<.0001
50 – 59 years	16.9%	20.0%	23.4%	146.26,	46.65,
				<.0001	<.0001
60 – 69 years	7.4%	16.8%	20.0%	1889.43,	43.92,
				<.0001	<.0001
70 – 79 years	4.2%	19.0%	20.5%	5261.07,	7.14,
				<.0001	0.01
80 years and older	3.6%	14.5%	15.1%	3579.83,	0.11,
				<.0001	0.71

(1) Veteran (as indicated on death certificate) compared to non-Veteran.
(2) Veteran with VHA service use compared to general population of Veterans. (as indicated on death certificate)

Additional information available from mortality records may help identify systematic differences among suicide decedents who were and were not identified as Veterans. Tables 6 – 8 show results from comparisons of non-Veterans, Veterans, and Veterans with history of VHA service use by marital status, race ethnicity, and educational attainment. Results from these comparisons are consistent with previous analyses of the characteristics of Veteran groups. Overall, suicide decedents identified as Veterans were more likely to have been married/widowed/divorced, be identified as non-Hispanic whites, and have comparatively higher levels of academic achievement.

Main Finding: Male Veterans who die by suicide are older than non-Veteran males.

Table 5. Percentage of Suicides by Age and Veteran Status among Females

Age Group	Non-Veteran	Veteran	VHA Veteran	, p (1)	, p (2)
29 years and younger	13.8%	12.9%	7.5%	3.31, 0.07	3.81, 0.06
30 – 39 years	17.3%	18.9%	13.5%	1.90, 0.17	2.13, 0.14
40 – 49 years	27.3%	34.1%	40.6%	19.78, <.0001	2.60, 0.11
50 – 59 years	21.7%	19.4%	24.1%	1.46, 0.23	1.45, 0.23
60 – 69 years	10.3%	7.1%	6.8%	7.77, 0.01	0.02, 0.90
70 – 79 years	5.6%	4.1%	2.3%	2.67, 0.10	1.47, 0.23
80 years and older	4.0%	3.5%	5.3%	0.41, 0.52	1.51, 0.22

(1) Veteran (as indicated on death certificate) compared to non-Veteran.

(2) Veteran with VHA service use compared to general population of Veterans. (as indicated on death certificate)

Main Finding: The age distribution of female Veterans and non-Veterans is similar.

Table 6. Percentage of Suicides by Marital and Veteran Status

Age Group	Non-Veteran	Veteran	VHA Veteran	, p (1)	, p (2)
Married/Separated	27.9%	38.6%	37.1%	1091.35, <.0001	65.96, <.0001
Widowed	4.8%	10.8%	11.1%	1225.35, <.0001	3.28, 0.07
Divorced	19.2%	22.1%	29.9%	105.31, <.0001	113.14, <.0001
Single	29.5%	11.5%	11.2%	3467.13, <.0001	7.97, 0.01
Unknown	18.6%	17.0%	10.7%	31.64 <.0001	11.24, 0.01

(1) Veteran (as indicated on death certificate) compared to non-Veteran.

(2) Veteran with VHA service use compared to general population of Veterans. (as indicated on death certificate)

Main Finding: Veterans who died from suicide were more likely to be married, widowed, or divorced.

Table 7. Percentage of Suicides by Race/Ethnicity and Veteran Status

Age Group Race	Non-Veteran	Veteran	, p
White	87.7%	92.6%	472.13,
			<.0001
African-American	6.4%	4.5%	128.55,
			<.0001
Indian/Native	1.6%	0.7%	122.17,
Alaskan			<.0001
Asian/Pacific	1.6%	0.4%	226.34,
Islander			<.0001
Other	0.7%	0.2%	89.39,
			<.0001
Unknown	2.0%	1.6%	10.01,
			0.01
Ethnicity			
Hispanic	5.4%	1.6%	676.81,
			<.0001
Non-Hispanic	87.2%	91.4%	351.21,
			<.0001
Unknown	7.4%	7.0%	6.61,
			0.05

Table 8. Percentage of Suicides by Education and Veteran Status

Age Group	Non-Veteran	Veteran	, p
Less than High	17.2%	10.3%	735.37,
School			<.0001
High School	30.8%	35.1%	174.36,
			<.0001
1 Year of College or	6.8%	7.9%	33.15,
Less			<.0001
2 Years of College	5.9%	7.0%	42.24,
			<.0001
3 Years of College	3.3%	3.5%	1.15,
			0.28
4 Years of College	7.5%	8.9%	56.24,
			<.0001
5+ Years of College	4.2%	5.1%	42.10,
			<.0001
Unknown	24.3%	22.2%	46.23,
			<.0001

Main Finding: The demographic characteristics of Veterans who have died from suicide are similar among those with and without history of VHA service use.

SUICIDE PREVENTION APPLICATIONS NETWORK/SUICIDE BEHAVIOR REPORTS

The VHA Strategic Plan for Suicide Prevention is grounded in a public health framework encompassing three major components: surveillance, identification of risk and protective factors, and development of effective prevention interventions. In accordance with the first component of this plan, surveillance, the VA has mandated since 2008 that health system facilities track attempted and completed suicides in a national database, the Suicide Prevention and Application Network (SPAN). Together, SPAN and the Department of Defense's Suicide Event Reporting system (DoDSER) which utilize the same standardized suicide event nomenclature constitute the nation's only real-time suicide surveillance systems. SPAN is coordinated and maintained by the Mental Health Program Director, Suicide Prevention and Community Engagement. The SPAN database compiles individual-level case reports for all suicide events and deaths known to VHA providers and Suicide Prevention Coordinators from each VHA medical facility using standard processes and a Suicide Behavior Report developed by national-level management and suicide prevention experts. VA policy requires that Suicide Prevention Coordinators complete a Suicide Behavior Report for all known suicides, suicide attempts, and some serious suicide ideation (i.e. suicide ideation involving a firearm). Therefore, reports of non-fatal suicide events may include suicide, suicide attempts and serious suicide ideation resulting in preventive action. In 2010, electronic reporting of suicide events was implemented.

The SPAN database provides the capacity for ongoing surveillance of suicide events among Veterans. Each month in FY2012, SPAN received approximately 1,400 suicide events nationwide, 95% of which are for non-fatal events. Although SPAN contains approximately 40% of suicide deaths among Veterans receiving VHA services, the State Mortality Data Project and annual all-cause National Death Index searches conducted for VHA users are better suited for tracking suicide deaths in the Veteran population. In contrast, SPAN is uniquely suited to capture information on the incidence and characteristics of non-fatal events. Furthermore, because SPAN is an internal data collection system, the SPAN system primarily contains suicide events for VHA utilizing Veterans; each year less than 10% of non-fatal suicide events reported to SPAN are for Veterans who are not recent VHA users. (VHA usually does not know about events for non-users).This report therefore focuses on non-fatal suicide events for VHA users defined as Veterans who have utilized any VHA services within one year preceding the event.

Prevalence and Characteristics of Non-Fatal Suicide Events

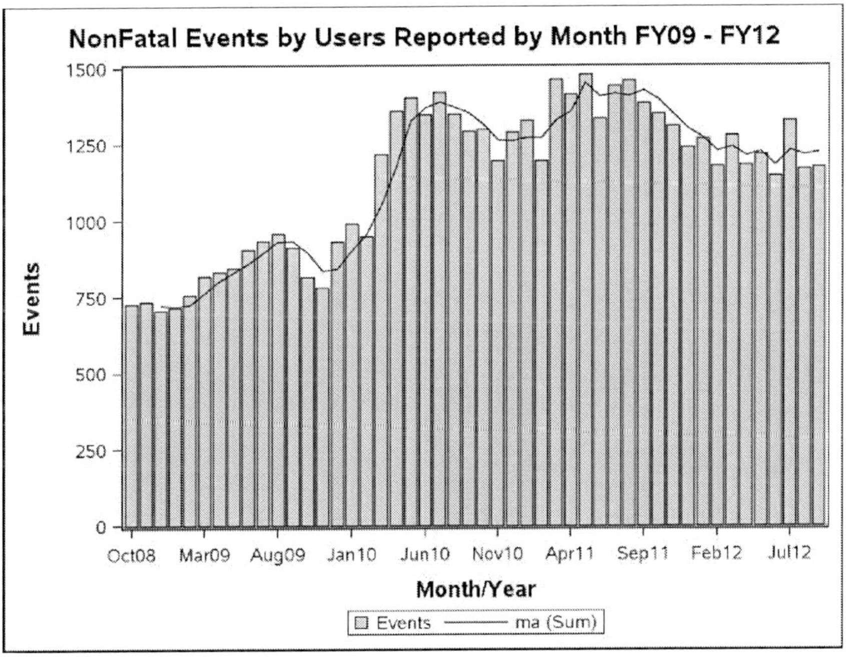

Figure 7. Number of Reported Suicide Events by Fiscal Year.

As shown in Figure 7, the absolute number of monthly non-fatal suicide events has increased since SPAN was implemented in 2008. However, early increases were likely due to a transitional period during which facilities were adapting to this new program and reporting procedures. The second period of the observed increase between December 2009 to July 2010 is likely due, in a large part, to the initiation of electronic submission of Suicide Behavior Reports, which streamlined the reporting process and potentially increased program compliance. There also appears to be a seasonal trend with more suicide events in the spring and summer months noted in 2010 and 2011. In the fall of 2011, the number of reported events again began to decrease, but the expected seasonal increase for the spring of 2012 was not observed. Thus, although findings are preliminary at this time, the number of non-fatal events appears to be decreasing. This observed decrease may represent a true decline in Veteran suicide behaviors, but could also be due, in part, to reporting lag or systematic policy changes regarding the types and number of events reported. This decrease is also observed when considering overall annual trends (Figure 8). In 2012, non-fatal suicide events were reported for almost 11,000 VHA users.

As some VHA utilizing Veterans experience multiple reported events, this corresponds to nearly 15,000 suicide suicide events reported in FY2012 compared to more than 16,000 in FY2011. This is unique data and cannot be compared to non-veteran data since population level non-fatal event data on the general population does not exist.

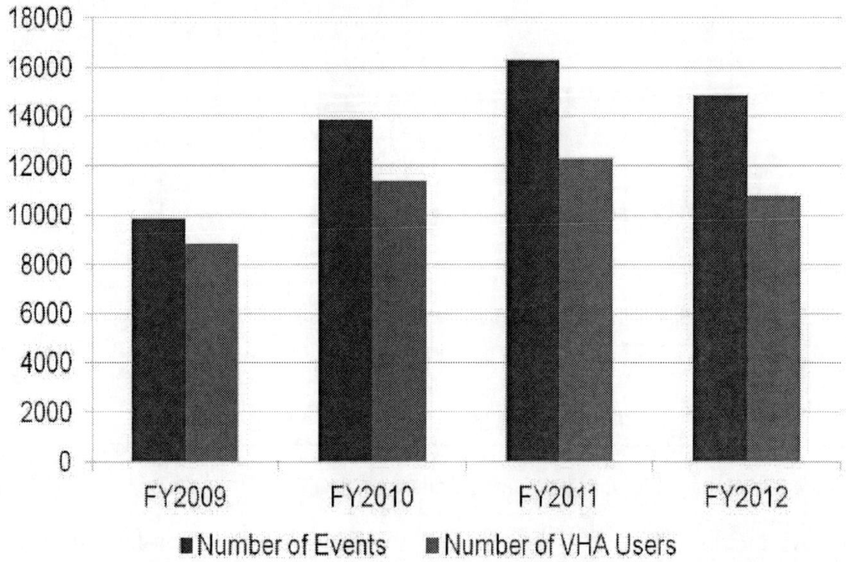

Figure 8. Number of Reported Suicide Events and VHA Users by Fiscal Year.

Main finding: Preliminary evidence suggests that the number of non-fatal suicide events for VHA utilizing Veterans has been decreasing since September, 2011.

Considering unique individuals with one or more non-fatal suicide events(s), the suicide event rate increased slightly from 2009 to 2011 and decreased slightly in 2012 parallel to that observed for the absolute number of events in figures 9 and 10. As shown in Figure 9, clear gender differences are apparent with more females than males with report of a suicide event each year, yet the annual trends are the same for both genders. Furthermore, the gender gap appears to be closing.

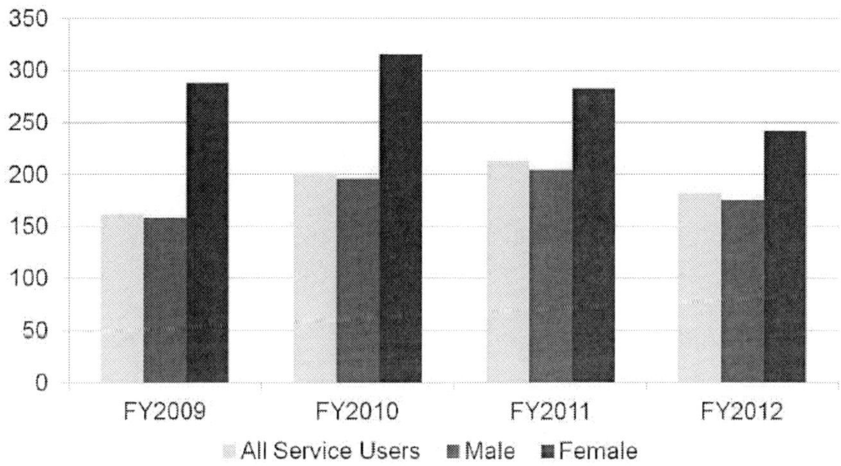

Figure 9. Rate of Non-Fatal Suicide Events by Sex and Fiscal Year.

Main Finding: Although gender differences exist, they appear to be decreasing.

Age-specific event rates clearly differ with a consistent patern emerging for 2009-2012. Rates are highest among younger Veterans and appear to decrease consistently with increasing age. Suicide event rates for Veterans 60 and older have remained comparatively stable since 2009, but fluctuations have been observed for younger Veterans. When considering rates by age group, we again see an increase from 2009-2010 for those less than 60 years of age, but a clear decline is noted beginning in 2011 and continuing in 2012. When considering Veterans of all ages, this decline was not apparent until 2012. This trend may be due to the fact that although rates are lower among older Veterans, there is a larger number of older Veterans utilizing VHA services and this group. Therefore, patterns in suicide event reports among older adults may disproportionately influence obseved trends in overall frequencies and suicide event rates. Among the older Veterans, no change in suicide event rates was observed between 2010 and 2011. Non-fatal event rates by age group and gender have been provided as Appendix C.

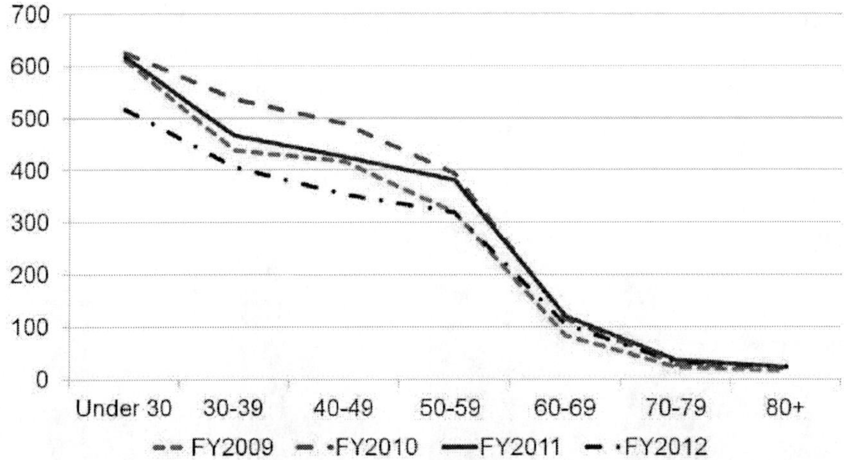

Main Finding: Rates of non-fatal suicide events decrease with age.

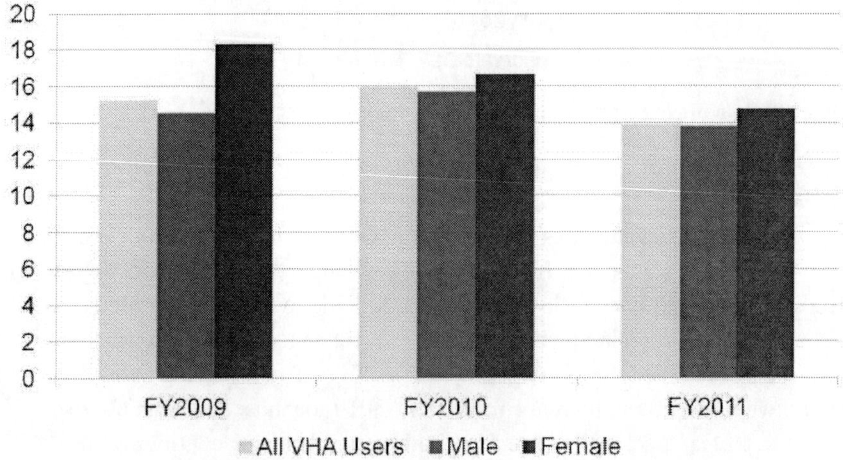

Figure 11. 12 Month Re-Event Prevalence by Sex and Fiscal Year.

Main Finding: The 12 month re-event prevalence decreased in FY2012.

Repeat report of an addiitonal suicide event within 12 months of a non-fatal sucide event occurs in approximately 15% of cases for both males and females. Although we cannot yet report on 2012 reattempt rates, it does appear that the 12 month repeat report prevalence decreased slightly from 2010 to 2011. Repeat report prevalence by age group and gender have been provided in Appendix D.

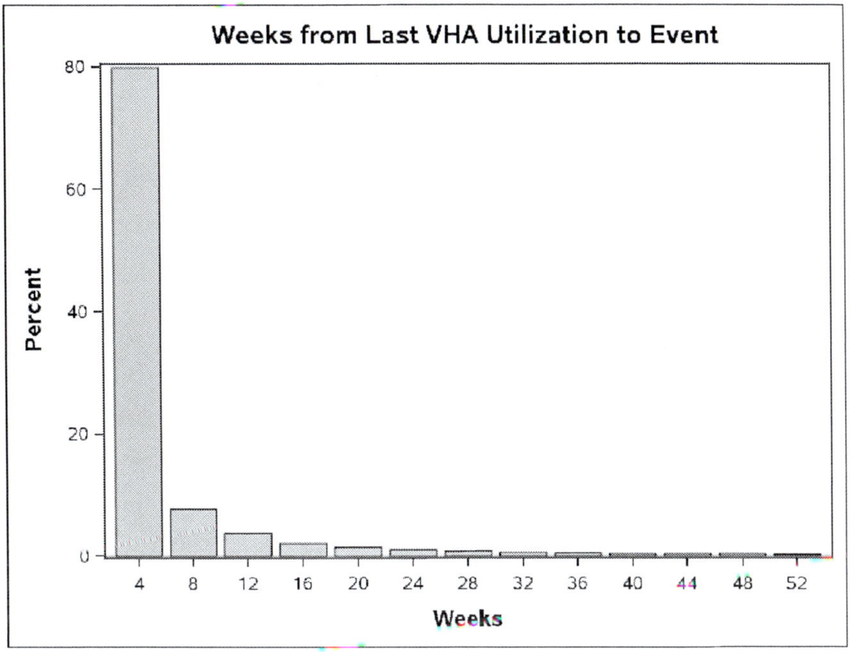

Figure 12. Prevalence of Non-Fatal Events by Time since Last Service Use.

Main Finding: Among those at risk, the first four weeks following service require intensive monitoring and case management.

Figure 12 clearly demonstrates that the majority (80%) of non-fatal events occur within four weeks of recieving VHA services. An additional 10% of events occur in the second month following last VHA service visit. These findings have important implications for treatment and prevention efforts as the majority of those with report of a suicide event are active, recent VHA users.

Furthermore, nearly 50% of the individuals with a VHA service visit in the year preeceeding the suicide event were last seen in the outpatient primary care setting (Figure 13). This implies that primary care should be an integral component of VHA suicide prevention programs and primary care clinicians should continue to receive support and training on the identification and management of those experiencing distress. Another 40% of those with report of one or more suicide events were last seen for mental health services indicating a need for continued assessment and risk management following use of VHA services among those with known risk factors (i.e. mental health diagnosis).

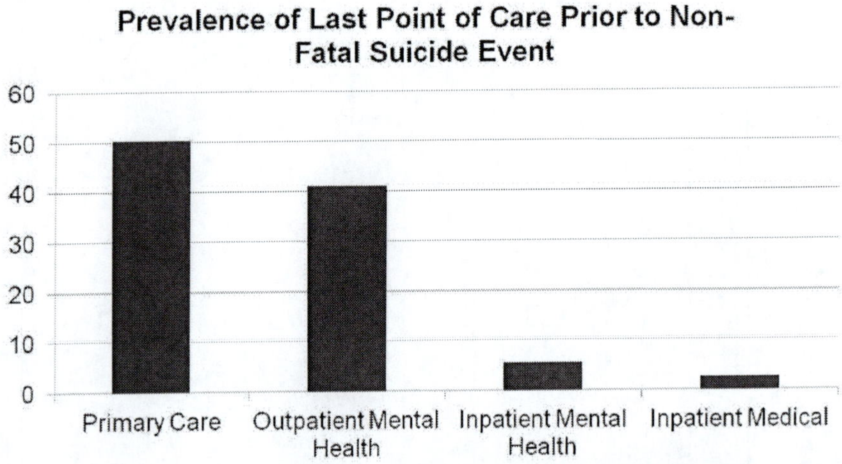

Figure 13. Prevalence of Last Point of Care Prior to a Non-Fatal Event.

Main Finding: The majority of Veterans who have a suicide event were last seen in an outpatient setting.

The majority of nonfatal events were the result of an overdose or intentional poisoning. However, nearly 11% of non-fatal attempts were made with a firearm. Additional research on the characteristics and outcomes among this group is needed. However, it is important to note that this number may include both Veterans who held a loaded gun but never discharged the firearm and those who suffered a non-fatal injury. Given the high case-fatality for firearm events in general, this finding highlights an opportunity and need to understand more about this group including risk factors, future suicide event rates and re-attempt methods in order to direct effective prevention and treatment services.

VETERANS CRISIS LINE

The Veteran Crisis Line application collects information related to calls from Veterans, their families and their friends in need. Calls are mainly

received from callers to the National Lifeline (1-800-273-TALK), where the caller pushed “1” for Veteran services. The Veteran Crisis Line is staffed 24 hours a day, 7 days a week by trained Veteran Affairs employees with backgrounds in mental health services. The information collected during each call includes date and time of call, history of suicidal ideation and events, access to means, substance use, social support, and perceived intent of suicide event. The majority of information is based on the flow of the call, and the number of mandatory fields is kept at a minimum. Most callers are anonymous (i.e. they do not provide identifying information) and do not result in a rescue. Information on outcome of the call and referrals for VHA services are collected and, when available, can be used to identify outcomes among callers to the Veterans Crisis Line (VCL).

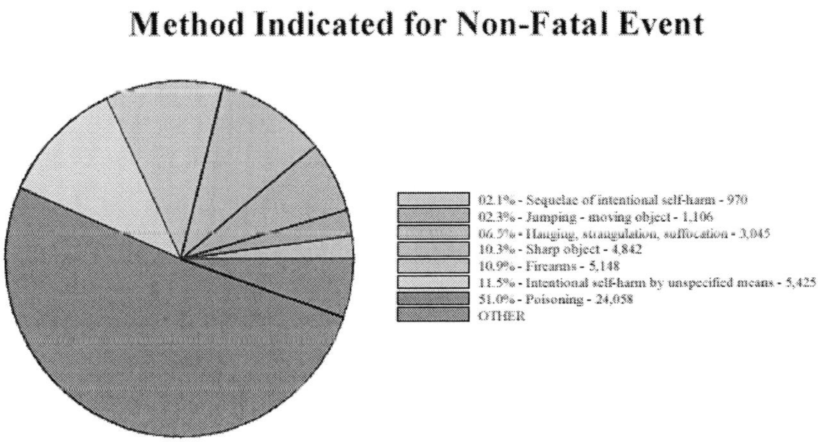

Figure 14. Prevalence of Method Indicated in Non-Fatal Event, FY2009-FY2012.

Main Finding: A majority of non-fatal events were the result or overdose or other intentional poisoning.

Prevalence and Characteristics of Calls to the Veterans Crisis Line

Since 2009, calls to the Veterans Crisis Line have continued to increase with a noticeable spike in call volume beginning in or around May 2011 (Figure 15). Around this same time, the VA re-branded the hotline from the

"Veterans Suicide Prevention Line" to the "Veterans Crisis Line" and launched the 'It's Your Call' media campaign promoting the newly named crisis line to Veterans and their family and friends. The evaluation of this campaign highlights this type of messaging as a viable method to encourage help seeking and promote the use of VA mental health services to Veteran populations. However, in order to support and sustain help seeking behaviors and maintain an upward trend in call volume the continuation of messaging activities should be considered.

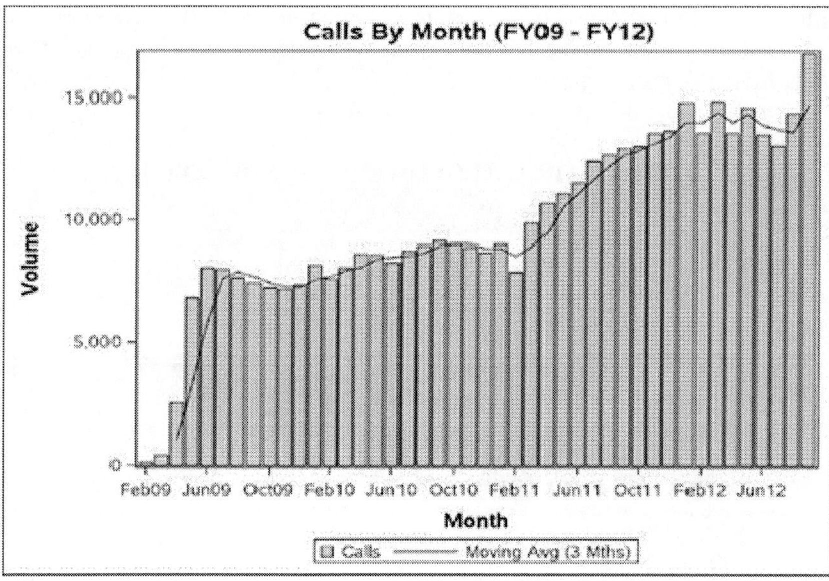

Figure 15. VCL Calls by Month.

Main Finding: Calls to the Veterans Crisis Line continue to increase and this increase may be associated with efforts to enhance awareness of VHA services through public education campaigns.

The percentage of repeat callers (i.e., callers from a single phone number or who have received a referral/rescue within 30 days of another call) has consistently increased over the past four years. For some, the Veterans Crisis Line may be instrumental in providing support and care and prompt individuals to access it more than once. As shown in Figure 16 below, the percentage of repeat callers has steadily increased over time from 17.25% in FY 2009 to almost 19.6% reported in FY 2012. These numbers may reflect change in the type of help individuals are seeking (e.g. rather than calling in crisis, calls may be for help with symptoms such as insomnia) or are indicative of the expansive role the Veterans Crisis Line may play in the provision of care to Veterans.

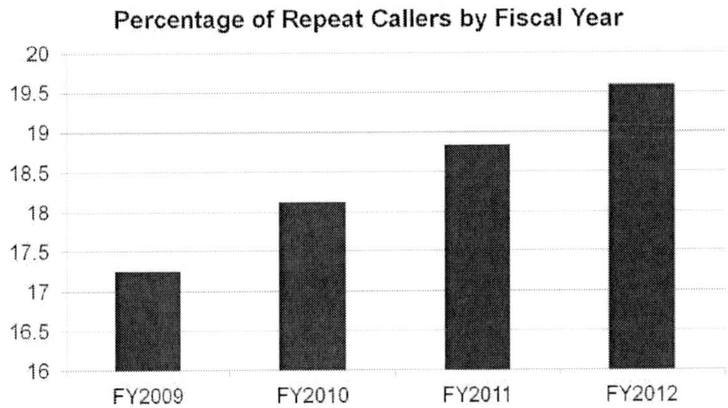

Figure 16. Percentage of Repeat Callers by Year.

Females accounted for approximately 20% of calls each month (Figure 17), however, the majority of callers to the Veterans Crisis Line were male (almost 80% per month). Despite identification as a group less willing to seek psychological help, males more often connected to the Veterans Crisis Line, a trend that was relatively stable between 2009 and 2012.

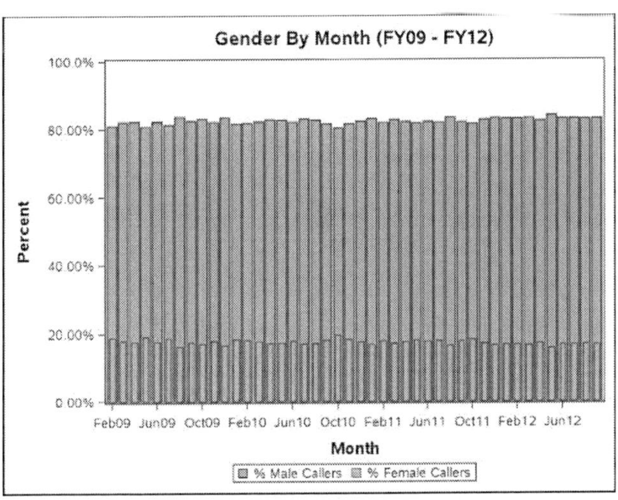

Figure 17. Percentage of Callers by Sex and Month.

Main Finding: The majority of all callers to the Veterans Crisis Line are male.

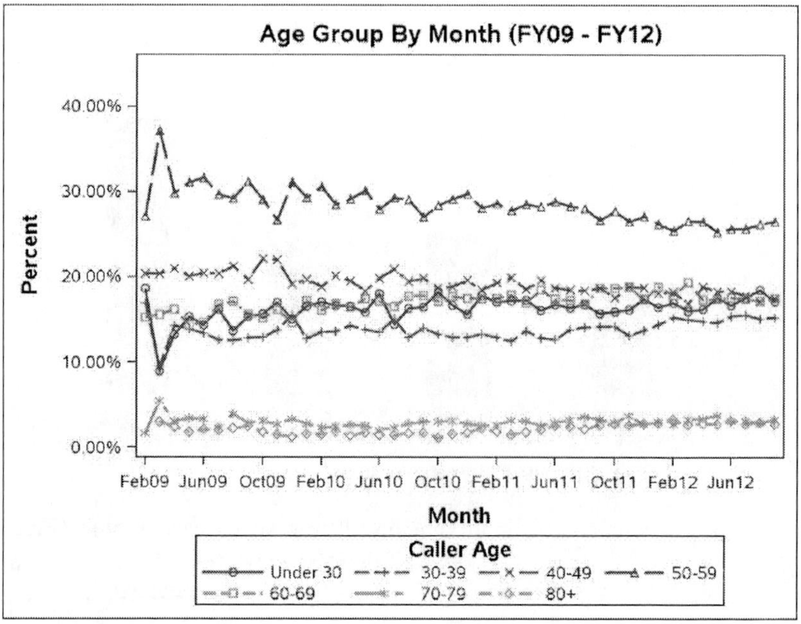

Figure 18. Percentage of Callers by Age Group and Month.

Main Finding: The majority of callers to the Veterans Crisis Line are between the ages of 50-59.

Although people of all ages utilize the Veterans Crisis Line, the largest percentage of calls each month to the Veterans Crisis Line were made by individuals between the ages 50-59 years old (approximately 30% of all calls each month).

Rates of suicide among middle-age men in the general population have increased during the past three years. Therefore, use of the Veterans Crisis Line may be particularly important for members of this group. As shown in Figure 18, the comparatively high prevalence of callers between the ages 50-59 years was sustained over time and suggests that the Veterans Crisis Line may provide a resource and access to care for those belonging to high-risk subgroups of the larger population. Overall, the percentage of calls to the Veterans Crisis Line from adults aged 40 years and younger and 60- 69 years is similar, with a comparatively small percentage (less than 10%) of calls among those aged 70 years and older.

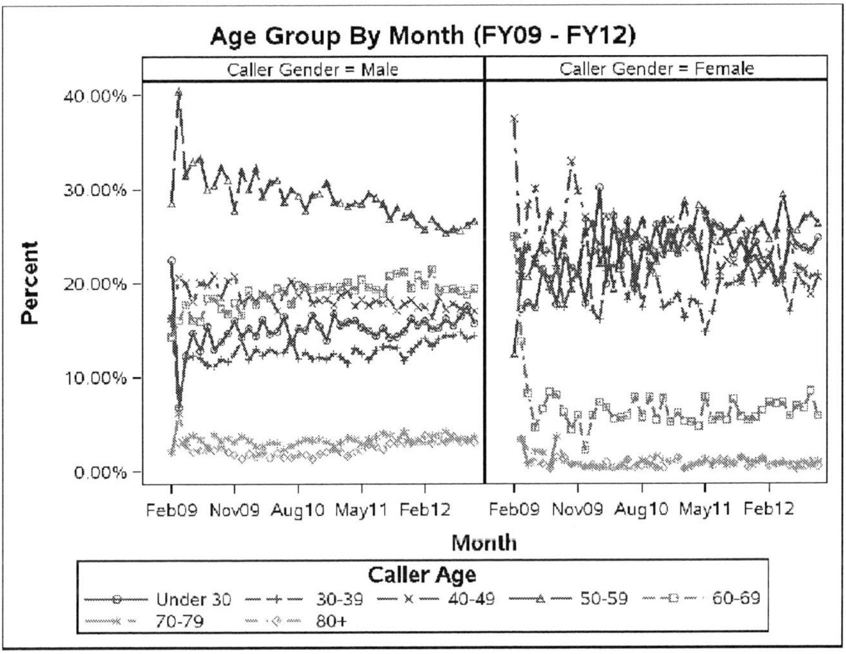

Figure 19. Percentage of Callers by Age Group, Gender, and Month.

Main Finding: Age composition of callers to the VCL is distinct between genders

Further analysis of monthly calls made to the Veterans Crisis Line reveal that the composition of callers' age differs by gender. The majority of male callers each month are between the ages of 50-59 with the fewest calls made by those ages 70 and older.

However, among female callers, the pattern is less distinct as trends in calls to the crisis line fluctuate over time with several age groups making the majority of calls (primarily those 59 and younger), and older females (70 and older) contributing less than 10% to calls per month.

A majority of all callers to the Veterans Crisis Line identified as Veterans (Figure 20). Overall, approximately 80% of all callers to the Veterans Crisis Line identify as Veterans and the remainder of other callers (including friends, family members, and all non-military others) contributed to less than 20% of total call volume each year.

The percentage of Veteran callers to the Veterans Crisis Line has remained comparatively constant since the first quarter of 2010. The sudden rise in Veteran callers from 60% in early 2009 to more than 80% in February

2010 may be attributable to a rebranding of the Veterans Crisis Line and the introduction of the Military Crisis Line in FY2011.

While the Veterans Crisis Line is identified to active duty personnel as the Military Crisis Line, the percentage of active duty callers has remained constant since February 2009 at just over 1%. It is possible that some active duty personnel may be identifying themselves as Veterans.

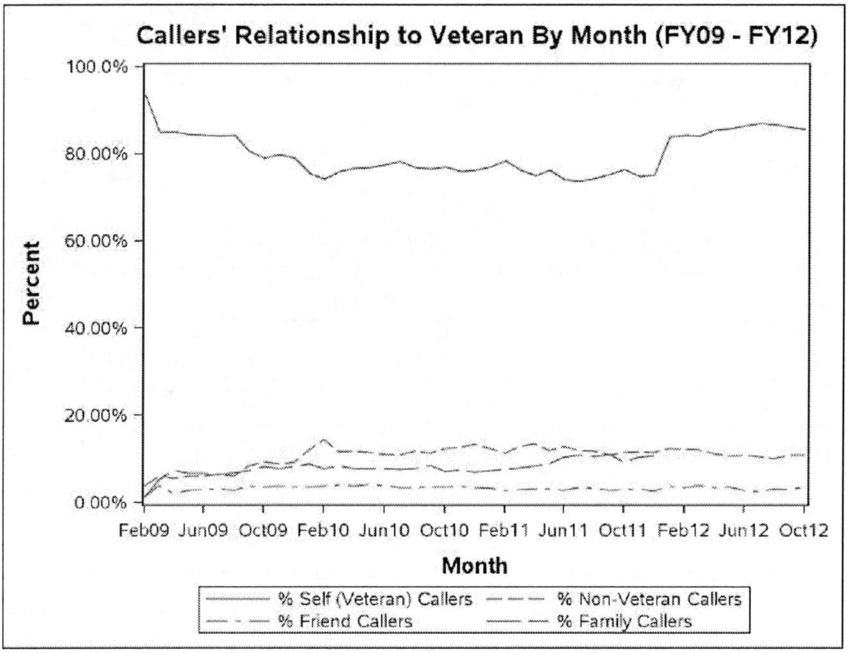

Figure 20. Relationship to Caller by Month.

Main Finding: Approximately 80% of callers to the Veterans Crisis Line identify as Veterans.

The percentage of repeat callers to the VCL has largely been relatively consistent across the past four fiscal years. (Figure 21)

However, a notable drop in the percentage of repeat callers is observable in early 2009, with the number of repeat callers falling from approximately 19% to 13%.

Since then, the percentage of repeat callers has continued to steadily increase back to approximately 19%, where is has remained fairly constant since the second quarter of 2011.

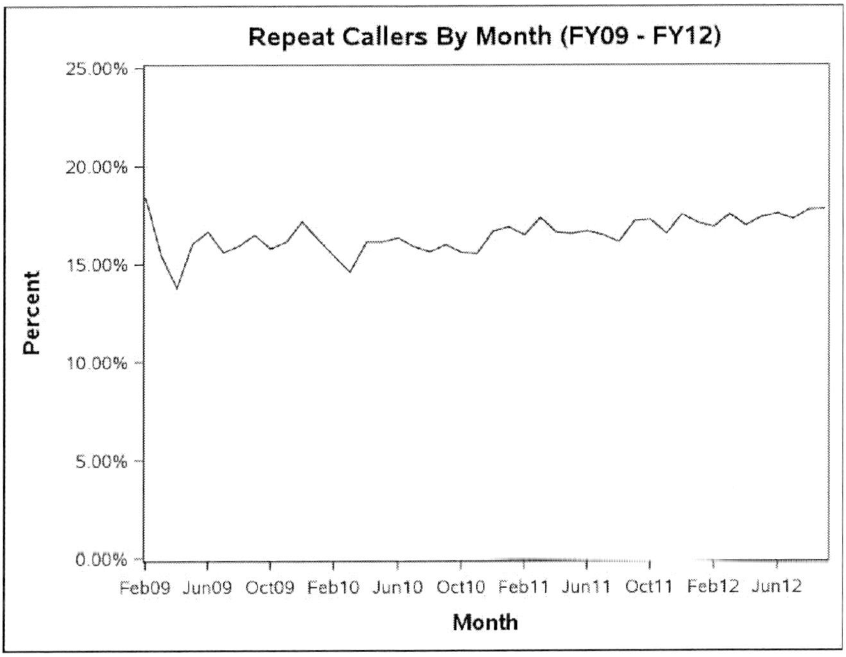

Figure 21. Percentage of Repeat Callers by Month.

Main Finding: Approximately 19% of calls to the Veterans Crisis Line call more than once each month.

Based on the prevalence of callers reporting thoughts of suicide at the time of the call, there currently seems to be a slight downward trend in the percentage of callers thinking of suicide (Figure 22). A sharp drop was first noted in early 2009, where this number fell from more than 40% to approximately 30%.

However, it is possible that this decrease was associated with implementation of the Veterans Crisis Line and characteristics of early adopters of this service.

This drop was then followed by a steady increase which peaked in the third quarter of 2010 at approximately 35%. This number has again decreased, with the percentage of callers thinking of suicide presently approximating to the same prevalence observed in 2009. Research is recommended to determine possible causes and differences in caller characteristics or outcomes associated with this change.

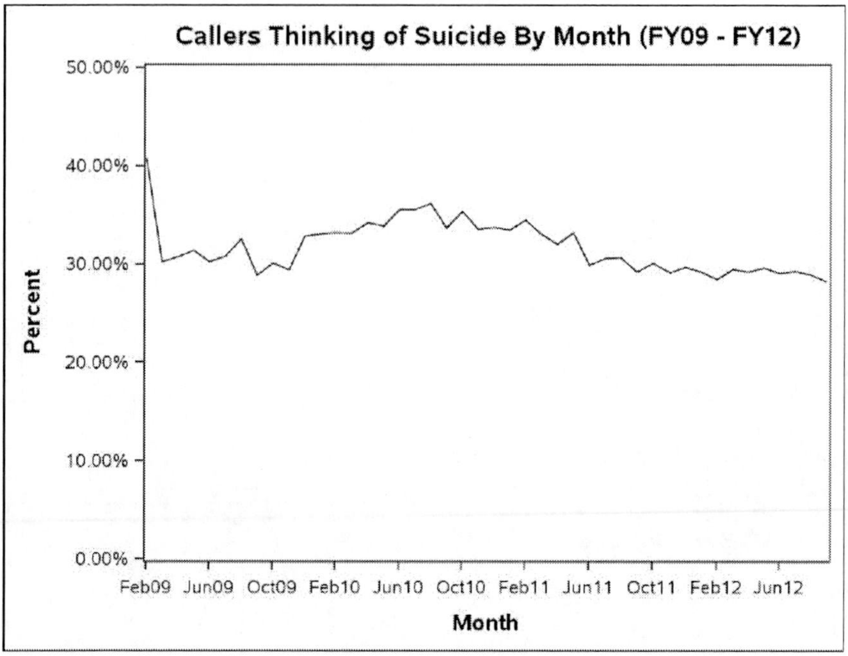

Figure 22. Percentage of Callers Thinking about Suicide by Month.

Main Finding: The percentage of callers to the Veterans Crisis Line who are currently thinking of suicide has decreased.

The number and percentage of rescues performed each month has also progressively declined (Figure 23).

Following a sharp drop in early 2009, this percentage of all calls resulting in a rescue increased to approximately 7% in June 2010 and has consistently decreased, now totaling approximately 3% of all calls. This change may be indicative of fewer callers presenting with crisis states making them at imminent risk of suicide as well as more callers presenting with a greater diversity of problems.

The percentage of callers receiving a referral has been steadily increasing from approximately 31% in early 2009 to more than 40% in FY2012 (Figure 24).

This increase may be due to callers to the VCL presenting more distally in the risk continuum or a shift in caller preferences, with more callers demonstrating willingness to accept referrals for clinical services.

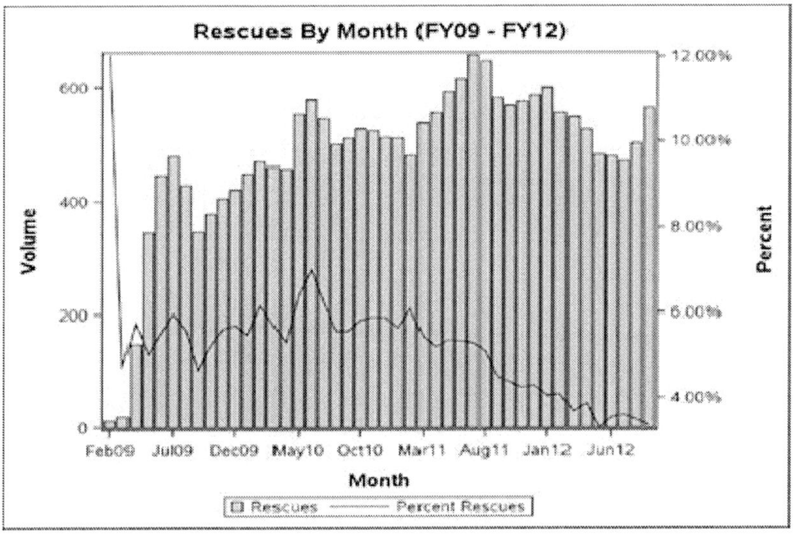

Figure 23. Number and Percentage of Rescues by Month.

Main Finding: The percentage of all calls resulting in a rescue has decreased.

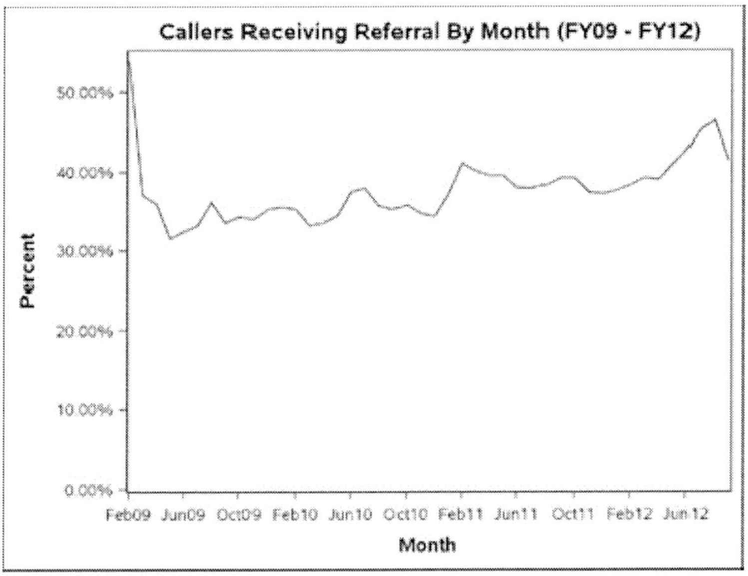

Figure 24. Percentage of Callers Receiving a Referral by Month.

Main Finding: The percentage of callers receiving a referral for follow-up care is increasing.

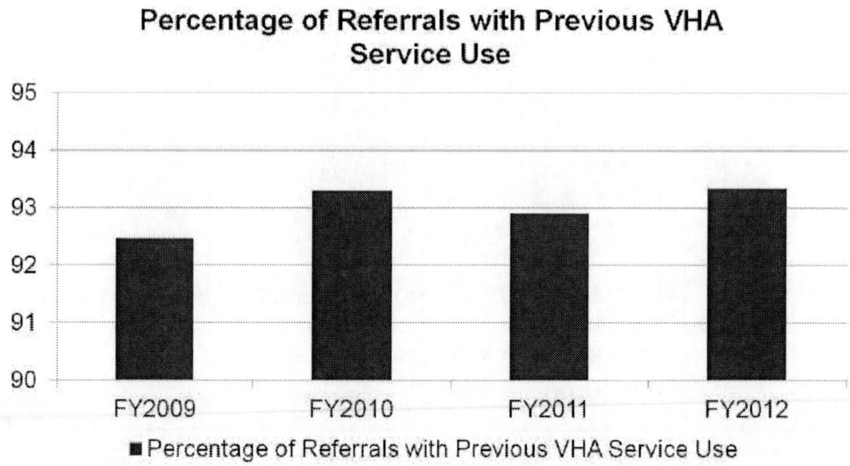

Figure 25. Percentage of Callers Receiving a Referral with Previous VHA Service Use by Month.

Main Finding: Approximately 93% of all Veterans Crisis Line referrals are made to callers with a history of VHA service use in the past 12 months.

The percentage of callers receiving a referral with history of VHA service in the 12 months preceding a referral rose from approximately 92.5% in FY2009 to just over 93% in FY2010 (Figure 25).

This number then slightly dropped in FY2011, only to return to just over 93% in FY2012.

Callers who receive more than one referral in a fiscal year have consistently between FY2009 – FY2012; with approximately 3% of all callers to the Veterans Crisis Line receiving more than one referral for care in FY2012 (Figure 26).

Figures 27-29 demonstrate patterns of VHA service use before and following a referral for service and are largely consistent across years. Between 61-90 days before the referral, mental health residential/domiciliary stays averaged 20 days per stay, decreasing to approximately 15 days per stay at 0-30 days after a referral. The length of a stay for residential and domiciliary care then increases to 22-23 days per stay at 61-90 days post-referral. In contrast, inpatient mental health stays averaged 7-8 days per stay at 61-90 days before and after a referral.

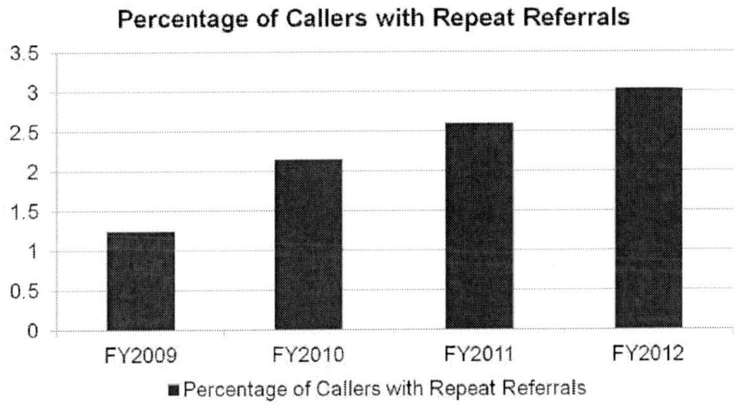

Figure 26. Percentage of Callers with Repeat Referrals by Year.

Main Finding: Slightly more than 3% of callers receive more than one referral each year.

Other inpatient stays slightly increased at 90 days following a referral, from approximately 5 days in FY2009 to 6-7 days in FY2010-FY2011. Other inpatient stays would then decrease to approximately 5 days per stay around the time of the referral, rising to 6-7 days per stay at 61-90 days after a referral. Overall, there was an average of 4 outpatient mental health encounters between 31-60 days after a referral, rising to an average of 5 encounters between 61-90 days following a referral.

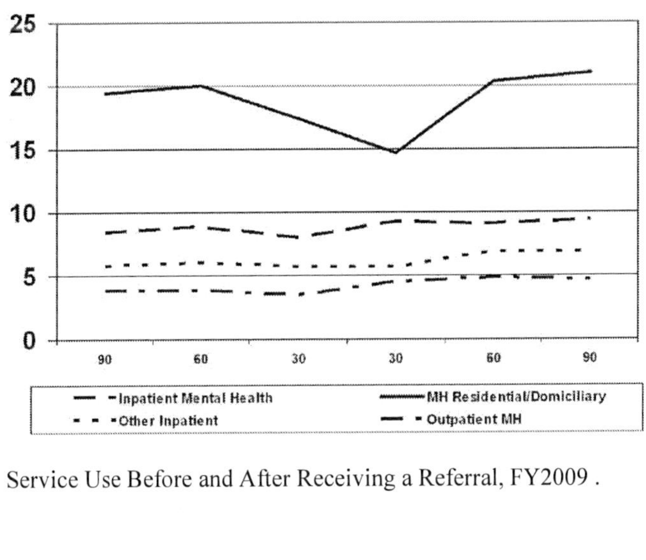

Figure 27. Service Use Before and After Receiving a Referral, FY2009 .

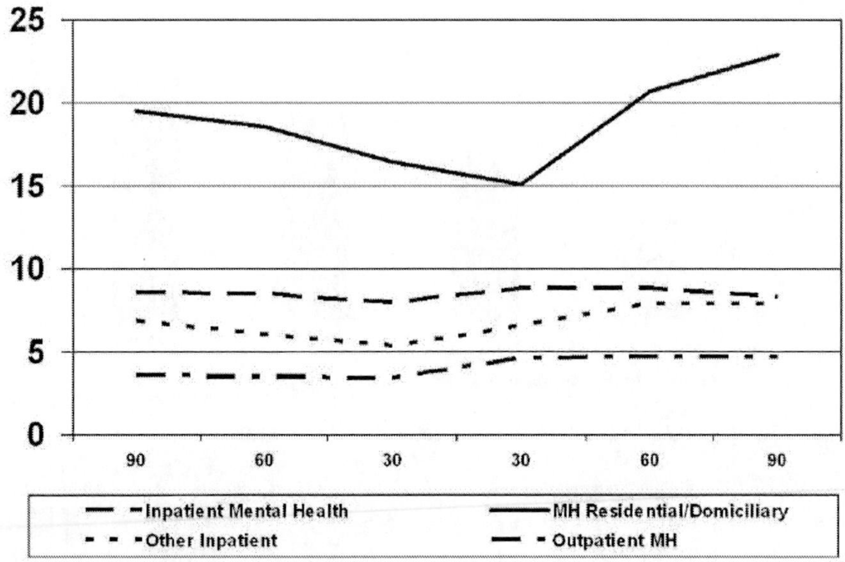

Figure 28. Service Use Before and After Receiving a Referral, FY2010.

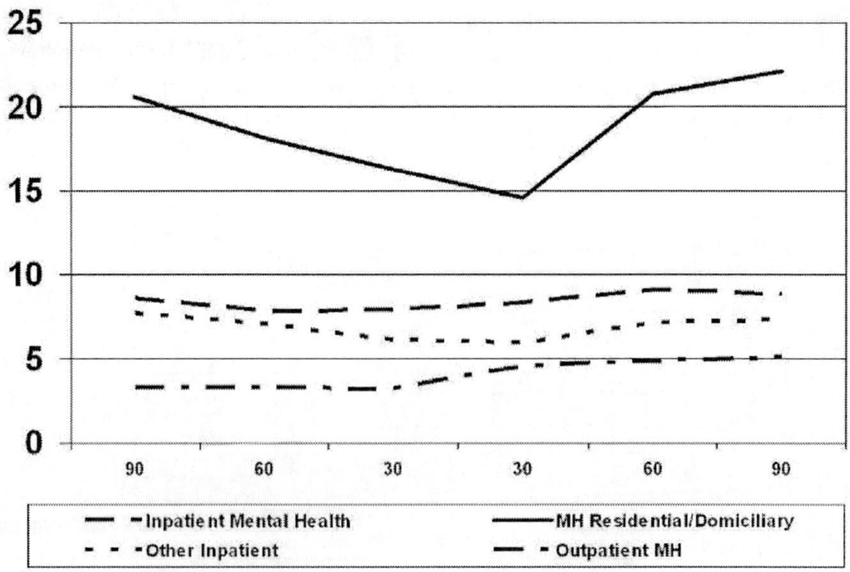

Figure 29. Service Use Before and After Receiving a Referral, FY2011.

Main Finding: Service use continues to increase following a referral for care.

Patterns of service use among Veterans with history of VHA services that were rescued following a call to the Veterans Crisis Line were consistent with increases noted following a referral. Overall, mental health residential/ domiciliary stays showed little variability between FY2010-FY2011, ranging from approximately 20 days per stay at 61-90 days before the rescue to 15 days per stay around the time of the rescue, rising to 21-22 days per stay at 61-90 days following a rescue (Figures 30-32).

The number of inpatient days and encounters varies from FY2009, where these stays rose to 25 days per stay at 1-30 days before a rescue, falling to 15 days in the 0-30 days following a rescue, rising to 20 days per stay at 61-90 days after the event. Between FY2009-FY2011, inpatient mental health stays averaged 8 days per stay at 30-90 days before the rescue, rising approximately 25% to about 10 inpatient days 31- 90 days after the rescue. Other inpatient stays averaged 6 days per stay at 31-90 days before and after the rescue in FY2009 and FY2011. In FY2010, other inpatient stays averaged 6 days per stay at 31-90 days before a rescue and rose to an average of 8 inpatient days between 61- 90 days after a rescue.

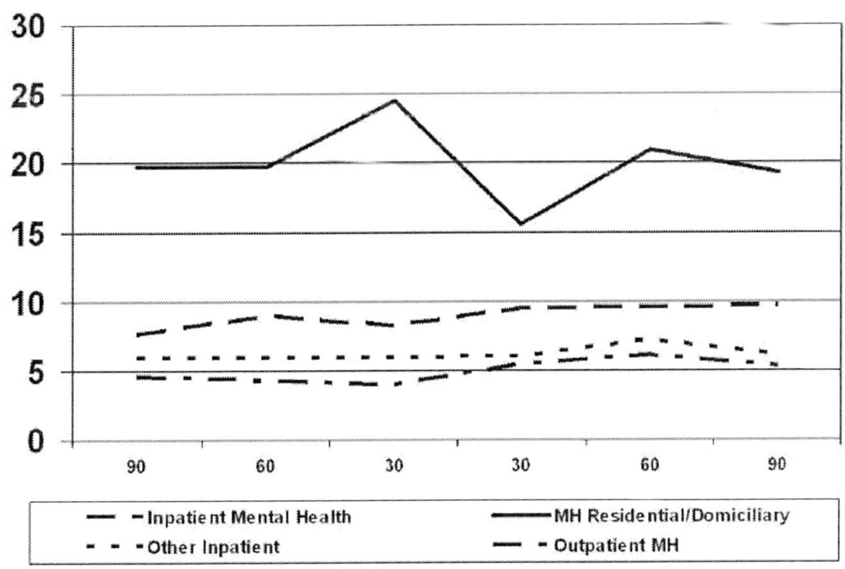

Figure 30. Service Use Before and After a Rescue, FY2009.

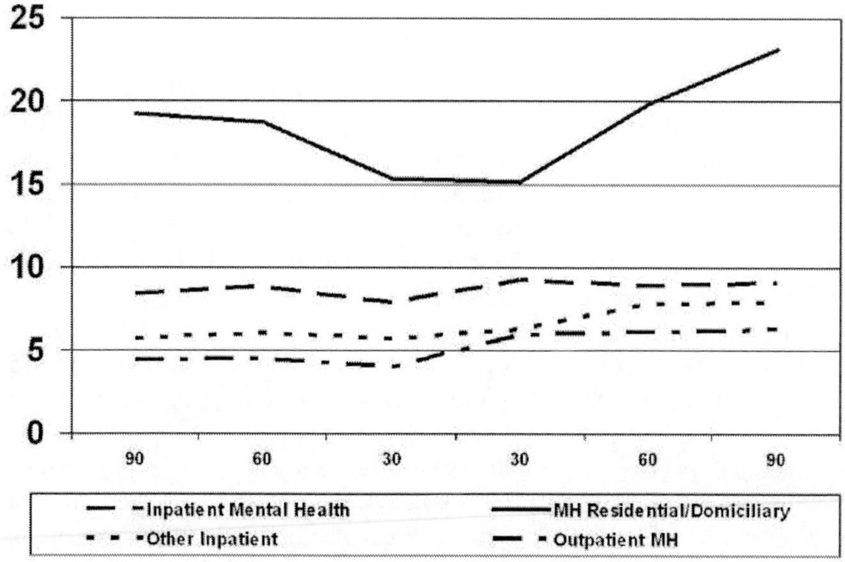

Figure 31. Service Use Before and After a Rescue, FY2010.

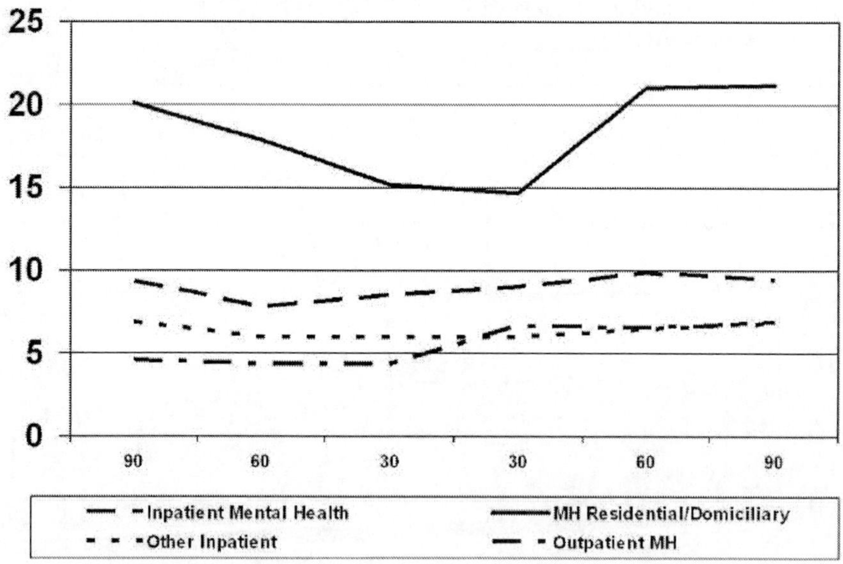

Figure 32. Service Use Before and After a Rescue, FY2011.

Main finding: Between FY2009 – FY2011, use of inpatient and outpatient services increased following a rescue.

Callers to the Veterans Crisis Line who receive a referral for follow-up care or who result in a rescue represent two groups that may be at increased risk for suicide. Increased risk for repeat suicide attempts has been identified among those who survive an initial suicide event and, among callers to the Veterans Crisis Line, may be greatest among Veterans who have attempted suicide before the time of their first referral or rescue resulting for a call to the Veterans Crisis Line. The suicide reattempt prevalence rate in FY2009 was approximately 19, increasing to 20 in FY2010, and decreasing to 18 in FY2011. (Figure 33) This change in 12- month reattempt prevalence rates may be due to a decrease in the number of non-fatal suicide attempters who call the Veterans Crisis Line as well as a sign of effective identification and management of risk following a rescue or referral.

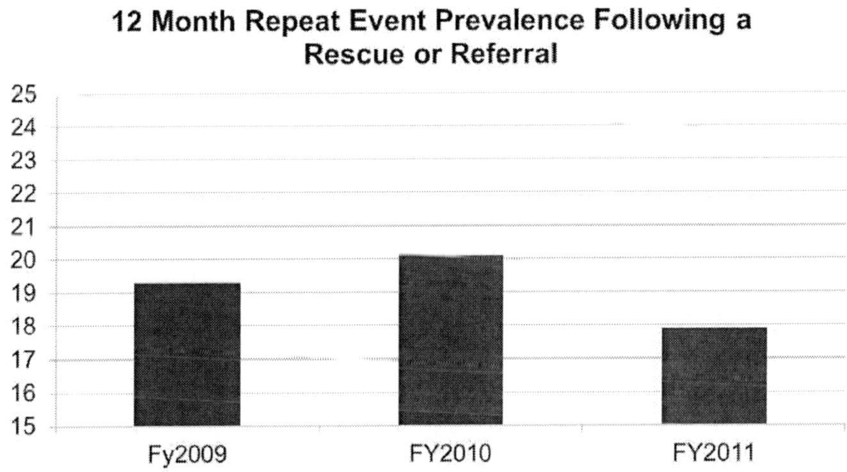

Figure 33. 12 Month Suicide Re-event Prevalence among Those Receiving a Referral or Rescue.

Main finding: The 12 month re-event prevalence has decreased among those who have been rescued or received a referral for follow-up care.

Conclusion

The report contains prevalence data and characteristics of suicide among Veterans and evidence of change in outcomes among Veterans at risk for suicide.

Included in this report are an overview and analysis of information collected through collaborative data sharing agreements with U.S. states, reports of non-fatal suicide events among Veterans using VHA services and analysis of data obtained from the Veterans Crisis Line. Data collected through the Department of Veterans Affairs' (VA) initiatives identify opportunities for the continued support and development of new prevention programs. Major findings of the report include:

- While the percentage of all suicides reported as Veterans has decreased, the number of suicides has increased
- A majority of Veteran suicides are among those age 50 years and older. Male Veterans who die by suicide are older than non-Veteran males who die by suicide.
- The age distribution of Veteran and non-Veteran women who have died from suicide is similar.
- The demographic characteristics of Veterans who have died from suicide are similar among those with and without a history of VHA service use.
- Among those at risk, the first 4 weeks following service require intensive monitoring and case management (which verifies the importance of the Enhanced Care Package for those at high risk).
- There is preliminary evidence in 2012 indicating a decrease in the rate of non-fatal suicide events for VHA utilizing Veterans.
- Decreasing rates of non-fatal suicide events are associated with increasing age.
- The data show a decrease in the 12 month re-event prevalence in fiscal year (FY) 2012.
- The majority of Veterans who have a suicide event were last seen in an outpatient setting. A high prevalence of non-fatal suicide events result from overdose or other intentional poisoning.
- Continued increases in calls to the Veterans Crisis Line may be associated with efforts to enhance awareness of VHA services through public education campaigns.
- The majority of callers to the Veterans Crisis Line are male and between the ages of 50- 59.
- Differences in the age composition of callers to the Veterans Crisis Line are associated with gender.

- A large percentage of callers to the Veterans Crisis Line are identified as Veterans.
- Approximately 19 percent of callers to the Veterans Crisis Line call more than once each month.
- The percentage of callers to the Veterans Crisis Line who are currently thinking of suicide has decreased.
- The percentage of all calls resulting in a rescue has decreased, indicating that the calls are less emergent and callers are using the Crisis Line earlier.
- The percentage of callers receiving a referral for follow-up care is increasing.
- Approximately 93 percent of all Veterans Crisis Line referrals are made to callers with a history of VHA service use in the past 12 months.
- Service use continues to increase following a referral for care.
- Between FY 2009 – FY 2011, use of inpatient and outpatient services increased following a rescue.
- The 12 month re-event prevalence has decreased among those who have been rescued or received a referral for follow-up care.

Although this was not a research-based analysis and there are significant limitations in the data that are available, as described in the report, this first attempt at a comprehensive review of Veteran suicide does provide us with valuable information for future directions in care and program development. While the numbers of Veterans who die from suicide each day has remained relatively stable over the past 12 years (varying from 18 -22 per day), the percentage of people who die by suicide in America who are Veterans has decreased slightly.

At the same time, the number of Americans who die by suicide each day has increased. This provides preliminary evidence that the programs initiated by VA are improving outcomes. VA must continue to provide a high level of care, and recognize that there is still much more work to do. As long as Veterans die by suicide, we must continue to improve and provide even better services and care.

This report provides us with valuable information about opportunities to do even better work.

A taskforce designed to provide recommendations for innovating Mental Health care in VA has been established and will be given this report to help guide its work.

A report from this interagency group will be forth-coming to the inter-agency task force developed to implement the Mental Health Executive Order which is highly focused on suicide prevention.

The work of this group includes developing action plans to address risk in a broader sense for all patients in both mental health and non-mental health settings.

This includes reassessing the value of traditional suicide risk assessments and screening (which is done now extensively in VA), and adding ways to identify life stressors and concerns earlier. Improving risk identification through these alternative approaches and increasing the numbers of Veterans who are engaged in the enhanced follow-up program may address that identified sensitive time period following VA contact as an outpatient as well as for inpatients.

Population groups indentified in the report that require additional interventions and engagement include women Veterans and Vietnam Era Veterans.

Additional VA training programs will be developed targeting providers of these groups of patients and Suicide Prevention Coordinators will be provided materials to do "refresher" training on suicide risk awareness and risk assessment for all staff.

Outreach remains critically important. Knowing that VA treatment strategies are effective provides an impetus to get more Veterans involved in treatment programs earlier.

Maintaining the availability of the Veterans Crisis Line to address all areas of concern for Veterans is valuable. Our communication and outreach strategies appear to be effective in this area – we should continue our work and expand in this area.

VA recognizes its role and responsibility in maintaining the safety and well-being of our nation's Veterans of all eras.

We will diligently continue to pursue successful and effective interventions for those Veterans at risk for suicide and those suffering from mental health related concerns through research and practice using all available information and data. We will continue to add to this information base as data continues to become available and provide updates to this on-going report.

APPENDIX A: VETERAN STATUS ON DEATH CERTIFICATE BY STATE AND YEAR

State/Year	1999	2000	2001	2002	2003	2004	2005	2006	2007	2008	2009	2010	2011
Alabama	K	K	K	K	K	K	K	K	K	K	K	K	K
Alaska	K	K	K	K	K	K	K	K	K	K	K	K	K
Arizona	A, NK	A, NK	A, NK	A, NK	A, NK	A, NK	A, NK	A, NK	A, NK	K	K	K	K
Arkansas	K	K	K	K	K	K	K	K	K	K	K	K	K
California	A,NK	A,NK	A,NK	A,NK	A,NK	A,NK	K	K	K	K	K	K	K
Colorado	K	K	K	K	K	K	K	K	K	K	K	K	K
Connecticut	A,NK	A,NK	K	K	K	K	K	K	K	K	K	K	K
Delaware	A,NK	A,NK	A,NK	A,NK	A,NK	A,NK	A,NK	A,NK	K	K	K	K	K
Florida	K	K	K	K	K	K	K	K	K	K	K	K	K
Georgia	A,NK	A,NK	A,NK	A,NK	A,NK	K	K	K	K	K	K	K	K
Hawaii	K	K	K	K	K	K	K	K	K	K	K	K	K
Idaho	K	K	K	K	K	K	K	K	K	K	K	K	K
Illinois	A,NK	A,NK	K	K	K	K	K	K	K	K	K	K	K
Indiana	K	K	K	K	K	K	K	K	K	K	K	K	K
Iowa	K	K	K	K	K	K	K	K	K	K	K	K	K
Kansas	K	K	K	K	K	K	K	K	K	K	K	K	K
Kentucky	A,NK	A,NK	A,NK	A,NK	A,NK	A,NK	A,NK	A,NK	A,NK	A,NK	A,NK	A,NK	K
Louisiana	K	K	K	K	K	K	K	K	K	K	K	K	K
Maine	K	K	K	K	K	K	K	K	K	K	K	K	K
Maryland	A, NK	A, NK	A, NK	A, NK	A, NK	A, NK	A, NK	A, NK	A, NK	A, NK	A, NK	A, NK	A, NK
Massachusetts	K	K	K	K	K	K	K	K	K	K	K	K	K
Michigan	K	K	K	K	K	K	K	K	K	K	K	K	K
Minnesota	K	K	K	K	K	K	K	K	K	K	K	K	K
Mississippi	A,NK	A,NK	A,NK	A,NK	A,NK	K	K	K	K	K	K	K	K
Missouri	K	K	K	K	K	K	K	K	K	K	K	K	K
Montana	K	K	K	K	K	K	K	K	K	K	K	K	K
Nebraska	A,NK	A,NK	A,NK	A,NK	A,NK	A,NK	K	K	K	K	K	K	K
Nevada	K	K	K	K	K	K	K	K	K	K	K	K	K
New Hampshire	K	K	K	K	K	K	K	K	K	K	K	K	K
New Jersey	K	K	K	K	K	K	K	K	K	K	K	K	K
New Mexico	A,NK	A,NK	A,NK	K	K	K	K	K	K	K	K	K	K
New York	K	K	K	K	K	K	K	K	K	K	K	K	K
New York City	K	K	K	K	K	K	K	K	K	K	K	K	K
North Carolina	A,NK	A,NK	A,NK	A,NK	A,NK	A,NK	A,NK	A,NK	A,NK	A,NK	A,NK	A,NK	A,NK
North Dakota	K	K	K	K	K	K	K	K	K	K	K	K	K
Ohio	K	K	K	K	K	K	K	K	K	K	K	K	K
Oklahoma	A,NK	A,NK	A,NK	A,NK	A,NK	A,NK	K	K	K	K	K	K	K
Oregon	K	K	K	K	K	K	K	K	K	K	K	K	K
Pennsylvania	K	K	K	K	K	K	K	K	K	K	K	K	K
Rhode Island	K	K	K	K	K	K	K	K	K	K	K	K	K
South Carolina	K	K	K	K	K	K	K	K	K	K	K	K	K
South Dakota	K	K	K	K	K	K	K	K	K	K	K	K	K
State Department	NA	NA	NA	NA	NA	NA	NA	NA	NA	NA	NA	NA	NA
Tennessee	A,NK	A,NK	A,NK	A,NK	A,NK	A,NK	A,NK	A,NK	A,NK	A,NK	K	K	K
Texas	K	K	K	K	K	K	K	K	K	K	K	K	K
Utah	K	K	K	K	K	K	K	K	K	K	K	K	K
Vermont	K	K	K	K	K	K	K	K	K	K	K	K	K
Virginia	K	K	K	K	K	K	K	K	K	K	K	K	K
Washington	K	K	K	K	K	K	K	K	K	K	K	K	K
Washington, DC	K	K	K	K	K	K	K	K	K	K	K	K	K
West Virginia	A,NK	A,NK	A,NK	A,NK	A,NK	A,NK	A,NK	A,NK	A,NK	A,NK	A,NK	A,NK	K
Wisconsin	K	K	K	K	K	K	K	K	K	K	K	K	K
Wyoming	A,NK	A,NK	A,NK	A,NK	A,NK	K	K	K	K	K	K	K	K

A=asked,
NA=not asked,
K=keyed,
NK=not keyed

Appendix B: Timeframe for Updated to Mortality Data by State

State	Timeframe of Data Availability
Alabama	Fall of following year
Alaska	Fall of following year
Arizona	Late Fall of following year
Arkansas	Spring of following year
California	Late Fall of following year
Colorado	Spring of following year
Connecticut	December of following year (last year finalized 2010)
Delaware	Late Fall of following year
Florida	Summer of following year
Georgia	Spring of following year
Hawaii	June of following year
Idaho	April 30th of following year
Illinois	Irregular, 2009 by Dec 2012, 2010 by Jan 2013, ongoing by 3rd Qtr
Indiana	Late Fall of following year
Iowa	June/July of following year
Kansas	Fall plus 1 year (last year finalized 2010)
Kentucky	Early Summer of following year
Louisiana	End of following year
Maine	June of following year
Maryland	Late Fall of following year
Massachusetts	Fall plus 3 years (last year finalized 2009)
Michigan	Late Summer/Fall of following year (2011 delayed due to new system)
Minnesota	Spring of following year
Mississippi	June of following year
Missouri	Late Spring/Early Summer of following year
Montana	Fall of following year
Nebraska	Fall plus 2 years (last year finalized 2010)
Nevada	Fall of following year
New Hampshire	Several Years behind in finalizing death files (last finalized 2007)
New Jersey	Fall of following year
New Mexico	June of following year
New York	Late Fall of following year
New York City	Late Fall of following year
North Carolina	Mid-Summer of following year
North Dakota	Fall of following year
Ohio	Spring of following year
Oklahoma	Several years behind in finalizing death files (last year finalized 2009)
Oregon	Summer plus 1 year (last year finalized 2010)

State	Timeframe of Data Availability
Pennsylvania	December of following year
Rhode Island	July 1 of following year
South Carolina	Late Fall of following year
South Dakota	May/June of following year
State Department	Ongoing
Tennessee	April/May of following year
Texas	December of following year
Utah	May/June of following year
Vermont	Winter plus 2 years (last year finalized 2009)
Virginia	Summer of following year
Washington	Fall of following year
Washington DC	July/August of following year
West Virginia	June of following year
Wisconsin	Jan/Feb of following year
Wyoming	June of following year

APPENDIX C: NON-FATAL EVENT RATES BY AGE GROUP AND GENDER (PER 100,000 USERS)

		2009			2010			2011			2012			FY09 - FY12	
		Unique Veterans With Event Report	Users	Rate Per 100,000	Unique Veterans With Event Report	Users	Rate Per 100,000	Unique Veterans With Event Report	Users	Rate Per 100,000	Unique Veterans With Event Report	Users	Rate Per 100,000	Unique Veterans With Event Report	Rate Per 100,000
	Total	8,823	5,440,000	161.06	11,377	5,638,263	201.78	12,309	5,795,165	212.40	10,764	5,896,509	182.55	43,273	189.98
	Under 30	1,311	214,387	611.51	1,551	247,840	625.81	1,804	291,978	617.85	1,579	305,135	517.48	6,245	580.52
	30-39	1,132	258,462	437.98	1,556	289,470	537.53	1,664	356,030	467.38	1,601	394,241	406.10	5,953	458.56
	40-49	1,918	459,153	417.73	2,405	489,755	491.06	2,337	548,441	426.12	1,960	554,337	353.58	8,620	420.14
	50-59	2,899	907,110	319.59	3,477	905,558	383.96	3,643	956,198	380.99	3,031	950,466	318.90	13,050	350.87
	60-69	1,208	1,461,232	82.67	1,865	1,620,883	115.06	2,137	1,775,373	120.37	1,893	1,829,412	103.48	7,103	106.22
	70-79	224	995,819	22.49	258	967,416	26.67	333	946,885	35.17	285	925,936	30.78	1,100	28.68
	80+	125	867,030	14.42	169	889,362	19.00	196	919,767	21.31	222	936,140	23.71	712	19.71
Male	Total	7,723	4,884,422	158.11	9,972	5,083,674	196.16	10,796	5,272,105	204.78	9,404	5,350,213	175.77	37,895	184.04
	Under 30	1,076	172,018	625.52	1,280	200,575	638.17	1,513	222,188	680.95	1,326	233,000	569.10	5,195	627.58
	30-39	881	206,209	427.24	1,257	231,201	543.68	1,319	266,438	495.05	1,285	296,161	433.89	4,742	474.20
	40-49	1,604	386,712	414.78	1,995	412,540	483.59	1,953	438,461	445.42	1,616	443,065	364.73	7,168	426.47
	50-59	2,645	823,474	321.20	3,147	810,801	388.13	3,261	813,122	401.05	2,703	803,176	336.54	11,756	361.66
	60-69	1,167	1,424,438	81.93	1,802	1,575,324	114.39	2,061	1,704,487	120.92	1,809	1,751,686	103.27	6,839	105.93
	70-79	222	981,144	22.63	243	951,938	25.53	322	928,182	34.69	277	906,783	30.55	1,064	28.24
	80+	123	847,219	14.52	162	869,672	18.63	191	899,227	21.24	216	916,342	23.57	692	19.59
Female	Total	1,089	377,872	288.19	1,279	405,385	315.50	1,479	522,567	283.03	1,318	545,454	241.63	5,165	279.00
	Under 30	232	40,364	574.77	233	47,265	492.97	278	69,790	398.34	237	72,135	328.55	980	426.91
	30-39	249	51,495	483.54	281	58,269	482.25	339	89,592	378.38	304	98,080	309.95	1,173	394.37
	40-49	314	71,610	438.49	383	77,215	496.02	377	109,980	342.79	336	111,272	301.96	1,410	381.00
	50-59	249	83,176	299.37	303	94,757	319.77	377	143,076	263.50	323	147,290	219.30	1,252	267.35
	60-69	40	36,527	109.51	55	45,559	120.72	74	70,886	104.39	84	77,726	108.07	253	109.67
	70-79	2	14,557	13.74	11	15,478	71.07	11	18,703	58.81	8	19,153	41.77	32	47.13
	80+	2	19,733	10.14	6	19,690	30.47	5	20,540	24.34	6	19,798	30.31	19	23.82

Appendix D: 12-Month Re-Event Prevalence by Age Group and Gender*

		2009			2010			2011		
		Total Count	Repeat Count	Percent	Total Count	Repeat Count	Percent	Total Count	Repeat Count	Percent
	Total	8,823	1,343	15.22%	11,377	1,816	15.96%	12,309	1,711	13.90%
	Under 30	1,311	174	13.27%	1,551	248	15.99%	1,804	238	13.19%
	30-39	1,132	189	16.70%	1,556	269	17.29%	1,664	220	13.22%
	40-49	1,918	279	14.55%	2,405	400	16.63%	2,337	342	14.63%
	50-59	2,899	477	16.45%	3,477	585	16.82%	3,643	576	15.81%
	60-69	1,208	178	14.74%	1,865	257	13.78%	2,137	256	11.98%
	70-79	224	25	11.16%	258	34	13.18%	333	38	11.41%
	80+	-	-	10.40%	-	-	6.51%	-	-	9.18%
Male	Total	7,723	1,123	14.54%	9,972	1,566	15.70%	10,796	1,492	13.82%
	Under 30	1,076	135	12.55%	1,280	199	15.55%	1,513	192	12.69%
	30-39	881	145	16.46%	1,257	212	16.87%	1,319	175	13.27%
	40-49	1,604	211	13.15%	1,995	327	16.39%	1,953	278	14.23%
	50-59	2,645	423	15.99%	3,147	528	16.78%	3,261	521	15.98%
	60-69	1,167	166	14.22%	1,802	249	13.82%	2,061	248	12.03%
	70-79	222	25	11.26%	243	31	12.76%	322	38	11.80%
	80+	-	-	10.57%	-	-	6.79%	-	-	9.42%
Female	Total	1,089	199	18.27%	1,279	213	16.65%	1,479	218	14.74%
	Under 30	232	34	14.66%	233	44	18.88%	278	46	16.55%
	30-39	249	40	16.06%	281	53	18.86%	339	45	13.27%
	40-49	314	62	19.75%	383	60	15.67%	377	63	16.71%
	50-59	249	51	20.48%	303	45	14.85%	377	55	14.59%
	60-69	-	-	25.00%	-	-	12.73%	-	-	10.81%
	70-79	-	.	.	-	-	18.18%	-	.	0.00%
	80+	-	.	.	-	.	.	-	.	0.00%

* Counts for groups with less than 20 events suppressed.

References

[1] Bahraini N, Gutierrez P, Harwood J et al. The Colorado Violent Death Reporting System (CVDRS): validity and utility of the Veteran status variable. Public Health Reports 2012; 127(3):304-309.

[2] Census. sex By age by veteran status for the civilian population 18 years and over. 2012. United States Census Bureau. 12-17-0012. Ref Type: Report.

[3] CDC. WISQARS. Web Based Interactive Statistical Query and Reporting System. 12-17- 0012. 12-17-0012. Ref Type: Electronic Citation.

In: Veteran Suicide
Editors: I. O. Walker and J. C. Gray
ISBN: 978-1-62618-548-7

Chapter 3

SUICIDE PREVENTION EFFORTS OF THE VETERANS HEALTH ADMINISTRATION*

Erin Bagalman

SUMMARY

Responsibility for prevention of veteran suicide lies primarily with the Veterans Health Administration (VHA), within the Department of Veterans Affairs (VA). The VHA Strategic Plan for Suicide Prevention is based on a public health framework, which has three major components: (1) surveillance, (2) risk and protective factors, and (3) prevention interventions.

No nationwide surveillance system exists for suicide among all veterans; therefore, the actual incidence of suicide among veterans is not known. Surveillance, or systematic collection of data on completed (i.e., fatal) suicides, is essential to define the scope of the problem (i.e., the suicide rate among veterans), identify characteristics associated with higher or lower risk of suicide, and track changes in the suicide rate over time to evaluate suicide prevention interventions. In the absence of a nationwide surveillance system for veteran suicide, the VHA is attempting to determine the rate of suicide among veterans in two ways,

* This is an edited, reformatted and augmented version of a Congressional Research Service publication, CRS Report for Congress R42340, from www.crs.gov, prepared for Members and Committees of Congress, dated January 10, 2013.

both in collaboration with the Centers for Disease Control and Prevention (CDC).

Information collected in surveillance is used to identify suicide risk factors (i.e., characteristics associated with higher rates of suicide) and protective factors (i.e., characteristics associated with lower rates of suicide). This is essential in order to design interventions that reduce risk factors and/or increase protective factors, thus lowering overall risk of suicide. Risk factors are also helpful in identifying at-risk groups or individuals so that interventions can be delivered to the people who need them most. Within the VHA, this research is supported by the Office of Research and Development; a Center of Excellence in suicide prevention; and a Mental Illness Research, Education, and Clinical Center on suicide prevention.

The intervention cycle includes three stages: design and test interventions, implement interventions, and evaluate interventions. The research components mentioned above have roles in small-scale pilot testing and large-scale evaluations of interventions. This report discusses seven areas of VHA suicide prevention interventions: (1) easy access to care, (2) education, (3) screening and treatment, (4) limited access to lethal means, (5) suicide hotline, (6) media restrictions, and (7) suicide prevention coordinators.

This report identifies challenges the VHA faces in each component of suicide prevention and discusses potential issues for Congress. A recurring theme is the need for the VHA to work in concert with other federal, state, and local government agencies; private for-profit and not-forprofit health care providers; veterans, their families, and their communities; and other individuals or organizations that might be able to help. Specific challenges in surveillance include timeliness of data, accurate identification of decedents as veterans, and consistent classification of deaths as suicides. Challenges in risk and protective factors research include a need for more collaboration and dialogue among agencies involved in suicide prevention and across other areas of public health (because suicide has some of the same risk and protective factors as other public health problems). Challenges in VHA suicide prevention interventions also include the need for more collaboration and dialogue, as well as an apparent gap between policy and practice, and misperceptions about mental illness and mental health care.

INTRODUCTION

Congress has attempted to address the problem of suicide among veterans through legislation,[1] and the House and Senate Committees on Veterans' Affairs have conducted oversight hearings, both on prevention of veteran suicide specifically and on veteran mental health more broadly.[2] The actual number or rate of veteran suicides is not known, because no nationwide surveillance system for suicide among all veterans exists, but there is consensus that the number is too high. Responsibility for prevention of veteran suicide lies primarily with the Veterans Health Administration (VHA), within the Department of Veterans Affairs (VA). Such a challenging task, however, demands collaboration with other federal agencies, state and local governments, other organizations, communities, and individuals.

Prevention of suicide can be approached in two ways, which are not mutually exclusive.

The public health approach intervenes with populations (e.g., distributing educational materials about mental illness and mental health services), whereas the clinical approach intervenes with individuals (e.g., prescribing antidepressant medication to a person diagnosed with depression). The individual focus of the clinical approach limits its reach to those who access the health care system;[3] clinical interventions are necessary but not sufficient. If the goal is to reach a broader population, the public health approach is considered essential.

The public health approach provides the framework for two suicide prevention strategies that are referenced in this report. The National Strategy for Suicide Prevention[4] involves multiple federal departments, including the VA, Defense (DOD), and Education (ED), as well as several agencies within Health and Human Services (HHS).[5] The VHA Strategic Plan for Suicide Prevention[6] is a compilation of VHA activities related to suicide prevention. While this CRS report focuses on suicide prevention efforts of the VHA, activities of other entities are discussed as they relate to VHA activities. The textbox briefly discusses eligibility for, enrollment in, and use of VHA services. As noted in the textbox, the majority of veterans do not use VHA services. VHA efforts to increase access to care—and to prevent suicide among veterans who do not use VHA services—are discussed later in this report.

Who Is a Veteran? Eligibility for, Enrollment in, and Use of VA Health Care

The term "veteran" may refer broadly to anyone who has served in the Armed Forces, including those currently serving. In this report, a veteran is someone who has separated from military service following a period of active duty.

Although an individual may return to active duty following separation (a particular issue among National Guard and Reserve members who have been activated), current active duty servicemembers are not the focus of this report.

Three additional points may be made relative to veterans and VA health care services:

- Eligibility: Not all veterans are eligible for VA health care services (see http://www.va.gov/healthbenefits); Vet Centers (non-medical facilities that provide readjustment counseling services for veterans and their families) have their own eligibility criteria (see http://www. vetcenter. va.gov/Eligibility.asp).
- Enrollment: Not all eligible veterans enroll in VA health care services. The number of enrolled veterans in FY2011 was 8.6 million, which is 39% of the estimated veteran population of 22.2 million. As noted above, some veterans are not eligible for VA health care services; others may choose not to enroll for various reasons (e.g., they might have employer-sponsored health insurance or other sources of health care services).
- Use: Not all enrolled veterans actually use VA health care services. The number of veterans who received health care services in FY2011 was 5.6 million, which is 65% of the 8.6 million enrolled veterans, or 25% of the estimated veteran population of 22.2 million. Enrolled veterans may choose not to receive care for various reasons (e.g., they might not perceive a need for health care services).

Sources: Estimated number of veterans is from Department of Veterans Affairs, FY2013 Budget Submission, Summary Volume, Volume 1 of 4, pp. 1F-1; numbers of veterans enrolled using services are from Department of Veterans Affairs, FY2013 Budget Submission, Medical Programs and Information Technology Programs, Volume 2 of 4, 2012, pp. 1B-3. See also Health Care for Veterans: Answers to Frequently Asked Questions, by Sidath Viranga Panangala and Erin Bagalman.

The VHA has received both praise and criticism for its suicide prevention efforts and mental health services more generally. In 2010 the federally funded Suicide Prevention Resource Center, in collaboration with the non-profit Suicide Prevention Action Network, published a progress report on an earlier version (2001) of the National Strategy for Suicide Prevention; the progress report (hereinafter referred to as *Charting the Future*) praises VHA's suicide prevention practices and recommends disseminating them to the rest of the health care system.[7] *Charting the Future* describes the VHA as "one of the most vibrant forces in the U.S. suicide prevention movement, implementing multiple levels of innovation and state of the art interventions, backed up by a robust evaluation and research capacity."[8] In contrast, some congressional testimony has criticized VHA's suicide prevention efforts for inadequacies, such as barriers to accessing care and lack of evidence-based treatments for those who do access care.[9] A 2011 evaluation of VHA mental health services (not limited to suicide prevention efforts) by the Altarum Institute and RAND Health captures both sides of the argument, finding that VHA mental health care is generally at least as good as that of other health care systems, but that it "often does not meet implicit VA expectations."[10]

This report begins with a brief overview of the public health framework for suicide prevention. The three subsequent parts of the report correspond to the three major components of the public health framework: (1) suicide surveillance, (2) suicide risk factors and protective factors, and (3) suicide prevention interventions. The final section addresses potential issues for Congress.

The importance of collaboration and dialogue is a recurring theme across all components of the VHA's suicide prevention efforts. Surveillance requires collaboration to address timeliness of data, accurate identification of decedents as veterans, and consistent classification of deaths as suicides. Risk and protective factors research requires dialogue among agencies involved in suicide prevention and across other areas of public health (because suicide has some of the same risk and protective factors as other public health problems). Successful prevention interventions also require collaboration. Challenges in prevention interventions include an apparent gap between policy and practice, as well as misperceptions about mental illness and its treatment.

A Public Health Framework for Suicide Prevention

As noted previously, both the National Strategy for Suicide Prevention and the VHA Strategic Plan for Suicide Prevention are based on a public health framework. As illustrated in *Figure 1*, the framework has three major components: (1) surveillance, (2) risk and protective factors, and (3) prevention interventions. Suicide surveillance involves collecting data on completed (i.e., fatal) suicides in order to define the scope of the problem. Data collected in surveillance can be used to identify risk factors (i.e., characteristics associated with higher suicide risk) and protective factors (i.e., characteristics associated with lower suicide risk). Suicide prevention interventions aim to reduce risk factors and/or enhance protective factors that have been identified; interventions may target high-risk groups or individuals, identified based on known risk factors.

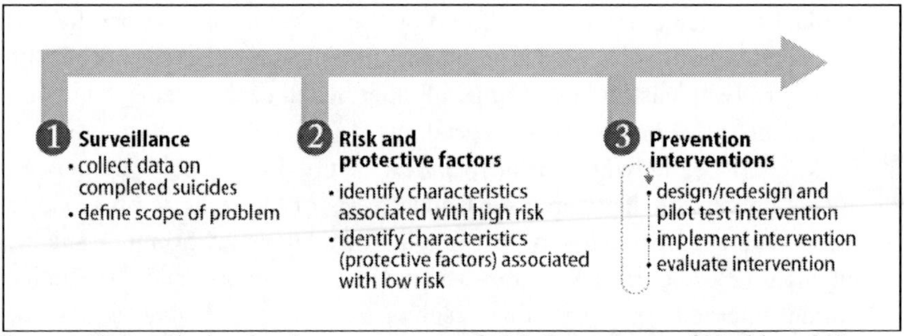

Source: CRS analysis of major components of U.S. Department of Health and Human Services (HHS) Office of the Surgeon General and National Action Alliance for Suicide Prevention, 2012 National Strategy for Suicide Prevention: Goals and Objectives for Action, Washington DC: HHS, September 2012.

Figure 1. A Public Health Framework for Suicide Prevention.

SUICIDE SURVEILLANCE

As noted previously, no nationwide surveillance system exists for suicide among all veterans. Surveillance, or systematic collection of data on completed (i.e., fatal) suicides, is essential for three purposes. First, surveillance defines the scope of the problem, that is, the suicide rate among veterans. Second, information from surveillance is used to identify characteristics associated with higher or lower risk of suicide. Third, information from surveillance is used to track changes in the suicide rate over time and evaluate suicide prevention interventions. In order to evaluate interventions, suicide surveillance must measure the same thing, in the same way, repeatedly over time.

In the absence of a nationwide surveillance system for veteran suicide, the VHA is attempting to determine the rate of suicide among veterans in two ways, both in collaboration with the Centers for Disease Control and Prevention (CDC). Combining the two methods provides more information about veteran suicide than either method alone, but the combination remains inadequate to the task. For example, one method is limited to enrolled veterans, and the other is limited to fewer than half the states; thus even the combination does not capture all veteran suicides. Also, statistics from both methods have a lag time of years, so that timeliness of data is an ongoing challenge. Each of the two methods is described below, along with its limitations and (where applicable) efforts to overcome those limitations.

Combining VHA Data with the National Death Index (NDI)

The VHA's primary approach to surveillance is illustrated in *Figure 2.* Information about completed (i.e., fatal) suicides is collected in death certificates by state, territorial, and local governments;[11] aggregated into the National Death Index (NDI) by the CDC;[12] and combined with enrollment data by the VHA in order to identify suicides among enrolled veterans.[13]

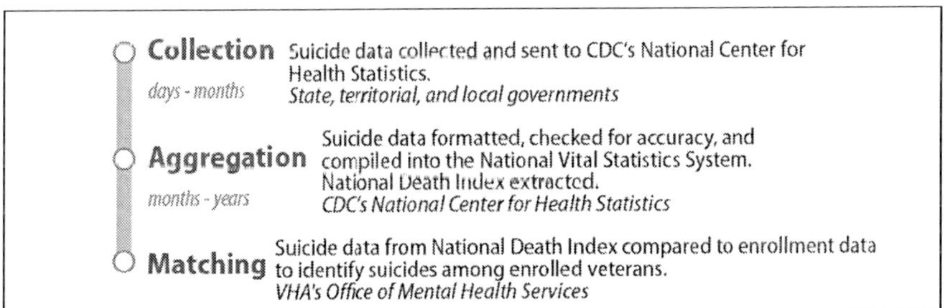

Source: CRS summary of information from CDC, National Center for Health Statistics, About the National Death Index, http://www.cdc.gov/nchs/data_access/ndi/about_ndi.htm; and from the VHA.

Figure 2. Combining VHA Data with the National Death Index.

This approach is subject to the following limitations:

- The resulting data may not be comparable across jurisdictions.[14]
- The lag between a suicide event and identification of the decedent as an enrolled veteran may be years; this delays the availability of crucial information.

- Suicides among non-enrolled veterans are not captured;[15] this leaves out the majority of veterans.[16]

Figure 3 presents annual suicide rates among VA-enrolled veterans. Suicide data are presented as rates to make them more meaningful (as opposed to a number of suicides without the size of the relevant population) and to make comparisons possible (e.g., across years or between genders). Annual suicide rates are commonly presented per 100,000 because the numbers would otherwise be extremely small (e.g., instead of 35.9 per 100,000 the number would be 0.000359).

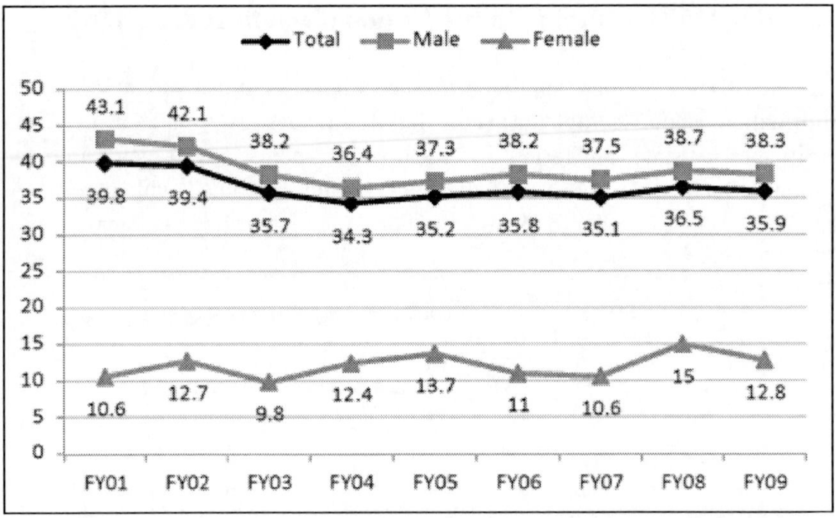

Source: CRS analysis of data provided by the Department of Veterans Affairs.

Notes: Rates are presented per 100,000 veterans enrolled in VA health care; for example, in FY2009, the rate of suicides was 35.9 per 100,000 veterans (male and female) enrolled in VA health care.

Figure 3. Annual Suicides per 100,000 VA-Enrolled Veterans, FY2001-FY2009.

Accessing the National Violent Death Reporting System (NVDRS)

In an attempt to identify suicides among veterans regardless of enrollment with the VA, the VHA uses the CDC's National Violent Death Reporting System (NVDRS), among other sources of information.[17] The NVDRS is a

CDC-funded program that enables participating states to supplement death certificates with information from law enforcement agencies, crime laboratories, coroner or medical examiner reports, health providers, and other state and local agencies. Through ongoing active surveillance, NVDRS may increase the likelihood that a death is recognized as a suicide and that a decedent's veteran status is captured (regardless of enrollment with the VHA). The CDC is working to address the limitations of this approach through the following activities:

- Expand the NVDRS to all 50 states, the District of Columbia, and the territories;[18] currently, the NVDRS is in operation in fewer than half the states.[19]
- Increase standardization of data collection and analysis, in order to increase comparability across states.[20]
- Assess the feasibility of linking VHA data directly to state NVDRS programs, thereby eliminating a step in the process and potentially reducing the lag time.[21]
- Link the NVDRS to data from the VHA and the DOD's Suicide Event Report, in order to increase accurate identification of veteran status.[22]

The timeliness of the data is a challenge for the VHA in both methods of surveillance described above. This is a challenge for suicide surveillance nationwide, not limited to suicide surveillance among veterans. Timely reporting of death certificates is identified as a core issue in the 2010 progress report on the earlier version (2001) of the National Strategy for Suicide Prevention.[23]

SUICIDE RISK FACTORS AND PROTECTIVE FACTORS

Identifying characteristics associated with higher rates of suicide (i.e., risk factors) and lower rates of suicide (i.e., protective factors) is essential in order to design effective interventions. Suicide prevention interventions aim to reduce risk factors and/or increase protective factors, thus lowering overall risk of suicide. Knowing what the risk factors are also helps in identifying at-risk groups or individuals so that interventions can be delivered to the people who need them most. Thus the second step in the public health framework for suicide prevention is identification of suicide risk and protective factors using data collected in surveillance. *Table 1* provides examples of risk and protective factors among the general population.

Table 1. Selected Risk and Protective Factors in the General Population

Risk Factors	Protective Factors
Some major physical illnesses, mental disorders, and substance use disorders	Effective clinical care for physical illnesses, mental disorders, and substance use disorders
Barriers to accessing health care	Easy access to a variety of clinical interventions
Stigma associated with help-seeking behavior	Support for help-seeking behavior
Easy access to lethal means (e.g., firearms or poison)	Restricted access to lethal means (e.g., firearms or poison)
Lack of social support and sense of isolation	Strong connections to family and community support
Cultural/religious beliefs that accept suicide	Cultural/religious beliefs that discourage suicide

Source: Examples of risk and protective factors selected from U.S. Department of Health and Human Services (HHS), Centers for Disease Control and Prevention (CDC), Injury Center: Violence Prevention, Suicide: Risk and Protective Factors, http://www.cdc.gov/violenceprevention/suicide/riskprotectivefactors.html.

Veteran-specific research on suicide risk and protective factors is necessary, because the veteran population differs from the non-veteran population on a variety of characteristics (e.g., gender distribution), some of which may also be associated with suicide risk. The subpopulation of veterans who are enrolled with the VHA may differ from non-enrolled veterans, as well.

The VHA conducts veteran-specific research that builds on research among the general population. Within HHS, both the CDC[24] and the National Institute of Mental Health (NIMH)[25] disseminate research on suicide risk and protective factors within the general population. Also, SAMHSA collects data on suicide attempts and related behavior.[26] It should be noted that risk factors for attempted suicide may differ from risk factors for completed suicide; for example, women have a higher rate of attempted suicide, but men have a higher rate of completed suicide.[27] Despite a large number of risk and protective factors identified by researchers, it is not yet possible to predict who will attempt or complete suicide.[28] The inability to identify individuals most in need of interventions is one of the reasons a public health approach—with a focus on population-level interventions—is necessary for effective suicide prevention.

Within the VHA, mental health research—including research on suicide risk and protective factors—is supported by two organizational units: the Office of Research and Development (ORD) and the Mental Health Strategic Healthcare Group (MHSHG). In general, the ORD funds intramural research by individual VHA investigators or researchers (including mental health care research).[29] The MHSHG funds a Center of Excellence (COE) in suicide prevention and a Mental Illness Research, Education, and Clinical Center (MIRECC) on suicide prevention, as well as centers addressing other mental health topics. Examples of research conducted on risk and protective factors by each of these three components—ORD, COE, and MIRECC—are provided below. The same three research components are also involved in the development and evaluation of suicide prevention interventions.

VHA Office of Research and Development (ORD)

The ORD's Health Services Research and Development Service supports research into suicide risk factors and protective factors.[30] For example, the VHA conducted a study to identify patient characteristics associated with higher suicide rates among veterans in treatment for depression (a known risk factor in the general population, as well as among veterans).[31] Another study examined characteristics associated with suicide risk among patients seen in VHA primary care, to help identify factors that primary care providers may be able to use to detect suicide risk.[32] These studies, and others like them, can help the VHA identify veterans at high risk of suicide, so that interventions can be targeted to them.

Center of Excellence (COE)

The COE at Canandaigua, NY, conducts research on suicide risk factors and protective factors, in addition to other suicide prevention activities. Established in August 2007 at the direction of Congress,[33] the COE has the mission of developing and studying evidence-based public health approaches to prevention of veteran suicide, with the goal of reducing morbidity and mortality associated with suicide in the veteran population. In pursuit of its mission, the Epidemiology and Interventions Research Core within the COE collects and analyzes data on suicide risk factors and protective factors (as well as other topics) among both veterans who use VHA services and those who do not.[34]

Mental Illness Research, Education, and Clinical Center (MIRECC)

The MIRECCs, also established at the direction of Congress,[35] conduct research on a range of mental health-related topics, including suicide risk factors and protective factors. Specifically, the MIRECC of the VA Rocky Mountain Network pursues the goal of reducing suicidality in the veteran population, by conducting research on potential contributions of cognitive and neurobiological factors, among other activities.[36] For example, one study assesses the relationship (if any) between prolonged grief and suicidal ideation.[37] Another study investigates the neurobiology of suicide risk in traumatic brain injury and substance abuse.[38] Other MIRECCs may also conduct research related to suicide, in the course of pursuing their other goals.

SUICIDE PREVENTION INTERVENTIONS

Through effective suicide prevention interventions, people's lives can be saved. Interventions aim to reduce risk factors and/or enhance protective factors, thereby lowering the risk of suicide. They may address entire populations (e.g., all veterans), at-risk subgroups (e.g., veterans diagnosed with PTSD), or high-risk individuals (e.g., veterans with recent suicide attempts).

Suicide prevention interventions are refined in a three-stage cycle. The first stage is to develop and pilot test interventions on a small scale to ensure that they are safe, ethical, feasible, efficacious (i.e., they work under ideal conditions), and effective (i.e., they work under real-world conditions). If interventions are successful in the first stage, the second stage is to implement them on a larger scale. The third stage is to evaluate interventions that have been implemented on a larger scale, to verify their effectiveness and determine for whom they are most effective. The three stages can then be repeated to refine interventions, either to improve their effectiveness or to adjust them for use with a different population (e.g., applying an intervention developed for male veterans to a population of female veterans).

Within the VHA, the same three research components involved in risk and protective factors research are involved in the intervention cycle: ORD,[39] COE,[40] and MIRECC.[41] Because small-scale testing and large-scale evaluation are both integral to suicide prevention interventions, it is worth noting that rigorous research on effectiveness is difficult and lacking for most interventions, both within and outside the VHA.[42]

The rest of this section discusses seven areas of VHA suicide prevention interventions: (1) easy access to care, (2) education, (3) screening and treatment, (4) limited access to lethal means, (5) suicide hotline, (6) media restrictions, and (7) suicide prevention coordinators.

Easy Access to Care

As noted previously, the majority of veterans do not use VHA services. Easy access to care is a protective factor against suicide,[43] and the VHA is making efforts to increase access to care by addressing identified barriers to care, including logistical challenges in scheduling or attending appointments, lack of understanding or awareness of mental health care, stigma associated with mental illness, and concerns about VHA care. In order to address these barriers, the VHA is taking two broad approaches: (1) increasing access to care by offering a broader range of mental health services (e.g., telehealth or off-hours clinics) and (2) providing education about mental illness and mental health care to veterans, their families, health care providers, and others in their communities.[44]

Offering expanded options in mental health services aims to alleviate logistical challenges by making services available in more places at more times.[45] VHA policy requires that new patients requesting or referred for mental health services receive an initial assessment within 24 hours and a full evaluation appointment within 14 days; follow-up appointments for established patients must occur within 30 days.[46] The extent to which these policies are implemented in practice has been questioned in congressional testimony, news media, and survey responses from both providers and patients.[47]

Educating veterans and others aims to increase understanding of mental health care and mental illness, reduce the associated stigma, and correct misconceptions about VHA care. For example, the VHA incorporates messages intended to reduce stigma into public health and outreach activities. In addition, the VHA is working to integrate mental health and substance use evaluation and treatment services into other treatment settings, which both increases the convenience and reduces the stigma associated with seeking care.[48] Educational interventions are described in more detail in the next subsection.

Education

The VHA offers suicide prevention education to audiences within VHA facilities and in surrounding communities. VHA requires suicide prevention training for all VHA staff that interact with veterans, plus additional training for health care providers. In the community, the VHA provides education for veterans' families and community "guides."[49] Community guides are trained to recognize individuals who may be at risk of suicide and help them seek treatment. Evidence supports education of guides; however, they must be able to refer individuals to quality mental health services.[50] Thus, access to care and quality of care are essential.

Screening and Treatment

Some types of screening, pharmacotherapy, and psychotherapy are supported by evidence that they reduce the likelihood of suicide.[51] VHA policy requires screening for a variety of risk factors, including depression, posttraumatic stress disorder (PTSD), problem drinking, traumatic brain injury (TBI), military sexual trauma (MST), and pain; veterans who screen positive must be offered follow-up evaluations and, if appropriate, treatment.[52]

An evaluation of VHA mental health care by the Altarum Institute and RAND Health finds that treatment in the VHA is generally better than in other systems on a variety of measures, but still has room for improvement.[53] In particular, the evaluation finds that evidence-based treatments (both pharmacotherapy and psychotherapy), while widely available, are not usually provided.[54] Researchers based this finding on a review of medical records, which showed that prescriptions for medication were often not filled for as long as recommended and that psychotherapy, as documented, was often not delivered according to evidence-based guidelines.

Additionally, the evaluation found that assessment is lacking, both at the beginning of treatment and during treatment (to track progress).[55] Even if a particular treatment is supported by evidence, it will not necessarily be effective for every patient. The only way to know whether a patient is improving, holding steady, or growing worse is to assess his or her symptoms at intervals.

Limited Access to Lethal Means

The three most common means of completing suicide among the general population are firearms (50%), suffocation (24%), and poisoning (18%).[56] Evidence supports restricting access to lethal means (e.g., firearms, gas, drugs) as a way to reduce suicide rates.[57] The VHA has a gun safety program (as both a child safety initiative and a suicide prevention initiative), which includes distribution of gun safety literature and gun locks. The VHA also encourages demonstration projects and research on blister packaging medications as a way to reduce the incidence of medication overdoses.[58] Means restriction is a promising area still under investigation.[59]

Suicide Hotline

Suicide hotlines are telephone numbers individuals can call for help in crisis situations (e.g., at the moment they are considering suicide). Hotlines are generally toll-free and available around the clock. The Veterans Crisis Line is a joint effort of the VHA and SAMHSA.[60] The main line (1- 800-273-8255) is the National Suicide Prevention Lifeline, operated by SAMHSA.[61] Veterans (or others calling with concerns about veterans) may select option 1 to be directed to the VHA's Veterans Crisis Line, answered by staff at the COE in Canandaigua, NY. Callers may remain anonymous or disclose their identify in order to allow the COE staff to access their VA medical records during the call. Since the Veterans Crisis Line began in 2007, it has received over 500,000 calls, resulting in over 73,000 referrals to Suicide Prevention Coordinators for same-day or next-day service. The Veterans Crisis Line is supplemented by an online chat service (http://www.VeteransCrisisLine.net/chat) and support via text messaging (text 838255).[62]

The evidence base for suicide hotlines is not sufficient to determine their effectiveness in reducing suicide rates, due to the difficulties inherent in conducting such evaluations.[63] The confidentiality of suicide hotlines renders follow-up with each individual caller impossible. Moreover, national hotlines, such as those operated by SAMHSA and the VHA, serve a large geographic area. A range of other interventions may be in place in localities within the hotline's reach, such that any change in the suicide rate may not be attributable to the hotline.

Media Restrictions

Exposure to a suicide—whether through a personal relationship with the decedent or through media coverage—is a risk factor for suicide.[64] In this way, suicide sometimes seems to act as a contagion, resulting in suicide clusters as one suicide is followed by other imitative suicides. Following a completed suicide, news media may restrict how suicides are reported (e.g., not glamorizing suicide or not reporting the specific means), in an effort to reduce the likelihood of imitative suicides. Evidence has shown that this may reduce suicide at a particular site (e.g., a bridge); however, more evidence is needed to determine whether this approach reduces the overall rate of suicide.[65] The VA monitors depictions of suicide in the media and (working with other federal agencies and partners in academia) encourages both news and entertainment media to depict suicide in a manner that is ethical and responsible.[66]

Suicide Prevention Coordinators

Per department policy, every VA Medical Center has at least one suicide prevention coordinator, whose responsibilities include (among other things) tracking patients who have been identified as at high risk for suicide; the VHA's computerized patient record system enables clinicians to flag high-risk patients, and policy requires that safety plans be developed for them.[67] A safety plan is a written document, developed jointly by a patient and a clinician, that identifies strategies for coping in a crisis (e.g., recognizing warning signs and contacting family members, friends, or mental health providers). Outside the VA, the use of suicide prevention coordinators has not been widely adopted, although some components of the program (e.g., safety plans) are widely used. The suicide prevention coordinator program has been identified as a practice worth emulating by a DOD task force on suicide prevention.[68]

Potential Issues for Congress

A recurring theme in recommendations regarding VHA suicide prevention efforts is the need for the VHA to work in concert with other federal, state, and local government agencies; private for-profit and not-for-profit health care providers; veterans, their families, and their communities; and other individuals or organizations that might be able to help. Specific recommendations are organized in the following subsections, according to the public health framework for suicide prevention: surveillance, risk and protective factors, and interventions. Public laws addressing suicide prevention among veterans are described in the *Appendix.*

Potential Issues in Surveillance

As discussed earlier, three challenges in suicide surveillance are (1) timeliness of data, (2) accurate identification of decedents as veterans, and (3) consistent classification of deaths as suicides. Addressing these three challenges requires the involvement of entities other than VHA.

The Center for a New American Security (CNAS)[69] offers three recommendations related to the timeliness of data. First, CNAS recommends that "Congress should establish reasonable time requirements for states to provide death data to the CDC."[70] It should be noted that states, territories, and cities voluntarily share vital statistics with the CDC. Congress may be able to facilitate or motivate more rapid data sharing by providing resources or incentives. Second, CNAS recommends ensuring that the CDC's ability to compile national death data expeditiously is not limited by a lack of resources.[71] Third, CNAS recommends that the annual analysis of veteran suicide data be coordinated among VA, DOD, and HHS.[72]

The VHA can identify decedents as veterans only if they are enrolled with the agency.[73] Identification of non-enrolled veterans relies on information gathered in the course of completing the death certificate or on supplemental information gathered as part of the National Violent Death Reporting System. VA researchers conducting a one-time study (not ongoing surveillance) combined information from the National Death Index with information from the DOD's Defense Manpower Data Center (DMDC) to identify suicides among veterans regardless of VA enrollment.[74] Congress may consider whether the DMDC is a source of information that can be used for suicide surveillance among veterans regardless of enrollment.

It is widely believed that inconsistent reporting of suicides across jurisdictions, as well as underreporting of suicides in general, limits the effectiveness of surveillance efforts.[75] Classification of a death as a suicide requires a determination that the death is both self-inflicted and intentional. Determining the decedent's intent is difficult, and coroners or medical examiners may feel pressure not to classify a death as suicide, due to the stigma associated with suicide. Suicides may be underreported when the manner of death is misclassified as "undetermined" or "accidental" (e.g., poisonings or single-vehicle crashes). Additionally, each jurisdiction (state, territory, or city) has its own requirements for investigating deaths, leading to variability across jurisdictions. Congress may be able to facilitate or motivate more standardization by providing resources or incentives.

Potential Issues in Risk and Protective Factors

Recommendations in the area of risk and protective factors include collaboration and dialogue both among agencies involved in suicide prevention and across other areas of public health. CNAS suggests information sharing between the VA, DOD, and HHS[76] and recommends that the House and Senate Committees on Veterans' Affairs initiate discussions with the House and Senate

Armed Services Committees to develop provisions addressing veteran suicide in the National Defense Authorization Act.[77] *Charting the Future* notes that suicide prevention tends to operate in its own silo, even though suicide has some of the same risk and protective factors as other public health problems. It recommends collaboration and dialogue between the suicide prevention effort and other public health efforts, stating, "Strong dialogue will help prevent the field from endlessly recreating wheels and spreading the limited funds too broadly to make a sustainable difference."[78]

Congress may choose to assess whether current levels of collaboration and dialogue are sufficient to ensure rapid dissemination of knowledge and avoid unnecessary duplication of effort. (Note that replication of studies is an integral part of the research process, so a distinction may be made between appropriate and unnecessary duplication of effort.) Congress may mandate, facilitate, or incentivize additional interagency coordination.

Potential Issues in Interventions

Three issues in VHA suicide prevention interventions that have come before Congress during hearings are (1) collaboration and dialogue, as discussed above; (2) an apparent gap between policy and practice; and (3) perceptions about mental illness and mental health care.[79]

If agencies (federal, state, or local) engage in ongoing collaboration and dialogue, sharing evaluations of existing interventions and research into new interventions, they may prevent unnecessary duplication of effort and help build the evidence base more quickly. The recommendations above regarding information sharing and collaboration pertain to intervention research as well.[80] *Charting the Future* advocates fast-tracking all phases of the intervention cycle (designing and pilot testing interventions, implementing interventions, and evaluating interventions), as well as the dissemination of the knowledge gained in each phase.[81] Moreover, congressional testimony has repeatedly called for increased use of non-VA resources, including other federal, state, and local government agencies; private for-profit and not-for-profit health care providers; veterans, their families, and their communities; and other individuals or organizations.[82] The use of non-VA resources might help suicide prevention interventions reach the majority of veterans who do not use VHA services.

A recurring theme in the area of suicide prevention interventions is the apparent gap between policy and practice. Examples of such a gap include the timeliness of mental health appointments and the use of evidence-based treatment. Increasing the timeliness of appointments may require congressional action in the form of additional resources in order to hire more providers, expand office space, or implement technologies such as telemedicine. Other gaps between policy and practice, such as the infrequent use of evidence-based treatment, may be possible for the VHA to address without additional resources; Congress may choose to continue exercising oversight in such areas.

Perceptions about mental illness and mental health care may affect whether veterans make use of treatment available to them. The belief that mental illness is a sign of weakness or something shameful may inhibit individuals or those around them from reaching out. Additionally, the belief that mental health care is not available, not appropriate, or not effective may discourage veterans from seeking care. Both stigma and mistaken beliefs may be reduced through discussions that address the facts of mental illness and mental health care. Thus congressional hearings on suicide, mental illness, or mental health care may have the unintended—but beneficial—consequence of reducing stigma and correcting misunderstandings about treatment.[83]

APPENDIX. PUBLIC LAWS ADDRESSING VA SUICIDE PREVENTION EFFORTS

Since Operations Enduring Freedom and Iraqi Freedom began, four public laws have addressed VHA suicide prevention efforts: the Joshua Omvig Veterans Suicide Prevention Act (P.L. 110- 110); the National Defense Authorization Act for Fiscal Year 2008 (P.L. 110-181); the Veterans' Benefits Improvement Act of 2008 (P.L. 110-389); and the Caregivers and Veterans Omnibus Health Services Act of 2010 (P.L. 111-163). Relevant provisions of each are summarized below.

Joshua Omvig Veterans Suicide Prevention Act

The Joshua Omvig Veterans Suicide Prevention Act (P.L. 110-110), enacted in 2007, required the VA Secretary to develop and implement a comprehensive suicide prevention program, and to report to Congress on the program. The Congressional Budget Office estimated that implementing the Joshua Omvig Veterans Suicide Prevention Act would have "little, if any, cost," because the VA already had implemented or was planning to implement each of the specific requirements.[84] The textbox below lists the required elements and additional authorized elements of the comprehensive suicide prevention program.

Joshua Omvig Veterans Suicide Prevention Act (P.L. 110-110)

Required elements of the comprehensive suicide prevention program include the following:

- mandatory suicide prevention training for appropriate VA staff and contractors;
- designation of a suicide prevention counselor at each VA medical center;
- outreach and education for veterans and their families to promote mental health;
- mental health assessments of veterans and referrals to appropriate treatment;
- availability of 24-hour mental health care for veterans;
- research on best practices for suicide prevention; and
- research on mental health among veterans with military sexual trauma.

Additional authorized (but not required) elements include the following:

- a 24-hour toll-free hotline staffed by trained mental health personnel;
- peer support counseling; and
- other actions to reduce the incidence of suicide among veterans.

National Defense Authorization Act for Fiscal Year 2008

Section 1611 of the National Defense Authorization Act for Fiscal Year 2008 (P.L. 110-181) directed the VA and DOD Secretaries to jointly develop a comprehensive care and transition policy for servicemembers recovering from serious injuries or illnesses related to their military service. The law specified that the policy must address (among other things) the training and skills of health care professionals, recovery coordinators, and case managers, to ensure that they are able to detect and report early warning signs of suicidal thoughts or behaviors, along with other behavioral health concerns. The law further specified that the policy must include tracking the notifications made by recovery care coordinators, medical care case managers, and nonmedical care managers to health care professionals regarding suicidal thoughts or behaviors, along with other behavioral health concerns. A 2009 Government Accountability Office report indicates that DOD and VA have developed the relevant policies.[85]

Veterans' Benefits Improvement Act of 2008

Section 809 of the Veterans' Benefits Improvement Act of 2008 (P.L. 110-389) grants the VA Secretary authority to advertise in the media for various purposes, including suicide prevention.

Caregivers and Veterans Omnibus Health Services Act of 2010

Section 403 of the Caregivers and Veterans Omnibus Health Services Act of 2010 (P.L. 111-163) requires the VA Secretary to conduct a study to determine the number of veterans who died by suicide between January 1, 1999, and May 5, 2010 (i.e., the date of enactment). As of this writing, the study has not been completed.

End Notes

[1] See the Appendix for public laws addressing suicide among veterans.

[2] See, for example, U.S. Congress, Senate Committee on Veterans' Affairs, VA Mental Health Care: Closing the Gaps, 112th Cong., 1st sess., July 14, 2011; U.S. Congress, Senate Committee on Veterans' Affairs, VA Mental Health Care: Addressing Wait Times and Access to Care, 112th Cong., 1st sess., November 30, 2011; U.S. Congress, House Committee on Veterans' Affairs, Subcommittee on Health, Understanding and Preventing Veteran Suicide, 112th Cong., 1st sess., December 2, 2011; and U.S. Congress, Senate Committee on Veterans' Affairs, VA Mental Health Care: Evaluating Access and Assessing Care, 112th Cong., 2nd sess., April 25, 2012.

[3] This report focuses on the public health approach. A full discussion of the clinical approach to suicide prevention is beyond the scope of this report. The pharmacotherapy and psychotherapy mentioned in the "Screening and Treatment" section are examples of the clinical approach.

[4] U.S. Department of Health and Human Services (HHS) Office of the Surgeon General and National Action Alliance for Suicide Prevention, 2012 National Strategy for Suicide Prevention: Goals and Objectives for Action, Washington DC: HHS, September 2012, http://www.surgeongeneral.gov/library/reports/national-strategy-suicide-prevention; hereinafter referred to as National Strategy for Suicide Prevention.

[5] Federal Working Group on Suicide Prevention, National Strategy for Suicide Prevention: Compendium of Federal Activities, 2009. HHS agencies involved in suicide prevention include the Centers for Disease Control and Prevention (CDC), Indian Health Service (IHS), National Institute of Mental Health (NIMH), Substance Abuse and Mental Health Services Administration (SAMHSA), Health Resources and Services Administration (HRSA), Agency for Healthcare Research and Quality (AHRQ), and Administration on Aging (AoA).

[6] Veterans Health Administration, VHA Strategic Plan for Suicide Prevention: FY 2009–2011; hereinafter referred to as VHA Strategic Plan. The VHA Strategic Plan is based on both public health and clinical approaches; see Element 2.1.

[7] Suicide Prevention Resource Center and Suicide Prevention Action Network (SPAN), Charting the Future of Suicide Prevention: A 2010 Progress Review of the National Strategy and Recommendations for the Decade Ahead, 2010, p. 18; hereinafter referred to as Charting the Future.

[8] Charting the Future, p. 11.

[9] See, for example, U.S. Congress, Senate Committee on Veterans' Affairs, VA Mental Health Care: Closing the Gaps, 112th Cong., 1st sess., July 14, 2011; U.S. Congress, Senate Committee on Veterans' Affairs, VA Mental Health Care: Addressing Wait Times and Access to Care, 112th Cong., 1st sess., November 30, 2011; U.S. Congress, House Committee on Veterans' Affairs, Subcommittee on Health, Understanding and Preventing Veteran Suicide, 112th Cong., 1st sess., December 2, 2011; and U.S. Congress, Senate Committee on Veterans' Affairs, VA Mental Health Care: Evaluating Access and Assessing Care, 112th Cong., 2nd sess., April 25, 2012.

[10] Katherine E. Watkins and Harold Alan Pincus, Veterans Health Administration Mental Health Program Evaluation: Capstone Report, Altarum Institute and RAND Health, 2011, p. 153; hereinafter referred to as VHA Mental Health Program Evaluation.

[11] Suicide surveillance relies on information derived from death certificates. Both the legal authority for maintaining registries of deaths and the responsibility for issuing death certificates reside with individual states, territories, and two cities (Washington, DC, and New York, NY).

[12] The National Center for Health Statistics (NCHS) is part of the Centers for Disease Control and Prevention (CDC), within the Department of Health and Human Services (HHS). NCHS works cooperatively with state, territorial, and local jurisdictions to collect information from death certificates in the National Vital Statistics System (NVSS). NCHS extracts information from NVSS to create the National Death Index (NDI), a data set that can be combined with other data sets for research purposes. For more information, see CDC, National Center for Health Statistics, About the National Death Index, http://www.cdc.gov/nchs/data_access/ndi/about_ndi.htm.

[13] VHA combines suicide data from the NDI with enrollment records to identify suicides among enrolled veterans. The enrollment file includes veterans receiving benefits from the Veterans Benefits Administration, even if the veterans are not receiving care from VHA.

[14] Researchers at the RAND Corporation summarized variation in suicide statistics across jurisdictions in four domains: (1) how suicides are defined or how ambiguous deaths are classified, (2) qualifications of professionals certifying a death as a suicide, (3) the extent to which possible suicide deaths are investigated, and (4) the quality of data management. Rajeev Ramchand et al., The War Within: Preventing Suicide in the U.S. Military, The RAND Corporation, 2011, p. 13, http://www.rand.org; hereinafter referred to as The War Within.

[15] The standard death certificate allows officials to indicate if a decedent has ever served in the U.S. Armed Forces; however, this indication captures both veterans and current servicemembers, with no means of distinguishing between the two. Also, the individual responsible for completing the death certificate may not know whether the decedent is a veteran.

[16] See textbox in the Introduction.

[17] VHA Strategic Plan, Element 7.1.

[18] HHS, CDC, Fiscal Year 2012 Justification of Estimates for Appropriation Committees. This goal is not reflected in the FY2013 Justification.

[19] HHS, CDC, National Violent Death Reporting System, http://www.cdc.gov/violenceprevention/nvdrs.

[20] HHS, CDC, Fiscal Year 2012 Justification of Estimates for Appropriation Committees. This goal is not reflected in the FY2012 Justification.

[21] HHS, CDC, National Center for Injury Prevention and Control, Division of Violence Prevention, Preventing Suicide: Program Activities Guide, Atlanta, GA, 2010.

[22] HHS, CDC, Preventing Suicide: Program Activities Guide.

[23] Charting the Future, p. 30.

[24] Centers for Disease Control and Prevention, Suicide: Risk and Protective Factors, Atlanta, GA, http://www.cdc.gov/ ViolencePrevention/suicide/riskprotectivefactors.html.

[25] HHS, National Institutes of Health (NIH), National Institute of Mental Health, Publications about Suicide Prevention, http://www.nimh.nih.gov/health/publications/suicide-prevention-listing.shtml; and National Institute of Mental Health, Science News about Suicide Prevention, http://www.nimh.nih.gov/science-news/science-news-aboutsuicide-prevention.shtml.

[26] SAMHSA asks about these topics in the National Survey on Drug Use and Health (NSDUH). See HHS, CDC, Morbidity and Mortality Weekly Report: Suicidal Thoughts and Behaviors Among Adults ≥ 18 Years—United States, 2008 – 2009, October 21, 2011, http://www.cdc.gov/mmwr/preview/mmwrhtml/ss6013a1.htm.

[27] HHS, Men's Health, Suicide, http://womenshealth.gov/mens-health/top-health-concerns-for-men/suicide.cfm.

[28] For example, although the single strongest predictor of a completed suicide is a prior suicide attempt, most people who attempt suicide do not subsequently complete suicide, and most people who complete suicides have no history of prior attempts. See The War Within and Joel Paris, "Predicting and Preventing Suicide: Do We Know Enough to Do Either?" Harvard Review of Psychiatry, vol. 14, no. 5 (2006), pp. 233-240.

[29] The ORD supports research through four research divisions: Biomedical Laboratory Research and Development (BLR&D), Clinical Science Research and Development (CSR&D), Rehabilitation Research and Development (RR&D), and Health Services Research and Development (HSR&D).

[30] A search for "suicide*" at http://www.hsrd.research.va.gov/research/ yields dozens of suicide-related studies conducted within ORD's Health Services Research and Development (HSR&D) Service; some of the resulting studies investigate risk factors and/or protective factors.

[31] VA, VHA, Health Services Research and Development, Suicide Among Veterans: Using the VA Depression Registry to Inform Care, Study IIR 04-211, http://www.hsrd.research.va.gov/research/abstracts.cfm?Project_ID=2141695453.

[32] VA, VHA, Health Services Research and Development, Suicidality: Correlates and Impact on Preference-Weighted Health Status of Veterans in VA Primary Care, Study SHP 08-160, http://www.hsrd.research.va.gov/research/ abstracts.cfm?Project_ID=2141698711.

[33] U.S. Congress, Committee of Conference, Making Appropriations for Military Quality of Life Functions of the Department of Defense, Military Construction, the Department of Veterans Affairs, and Related Agencies for the Fiscal Year Ending September 30, 2006, and for Other Purposes, report to accompany H.R. 2528, 109th Cong., 1st sess., November 18, 2005, H.Rept. 109-305 (Washington: GPO, 2006), p. 39. The committee report directed the VHA "to place more emphasis on psychiatric care of our veterans by designating three

centers of excellence to focus on mental health/PTSD needs. These three centers will be established at Waco Medical Center, Texas; San Diego Medical Center, California; and the Canandaigua Medical Center, New York."

[34] VA, VHA, VISN 2 Center of Excellence at Canandaigua, http://www.mirecc.va.gov/docs/ 2010InfoSheets/ VISN_2_CoE_Canandaigua_Info_Sheet_2010.pdf.

[35] P.L. 104-262, Veterans' Health Care Eligibility Reform Act of 1996, enacted 10/09/1996 (38 U.S.C. §7320).

[36] VA, VHA, MIRECC of the VA Rocky Mountain Network (VISN 19 MIRECC), http://www.mirecc.va.gov/visn19/ index.asp.

[37] VA, VHA, VISN 19 MIRECC, Examining Prolonged Grief Disorder and Its Relationship to Self-Directed Violence (SDV) Among Veterans, http://www.mirecc.va.gov/visn19/ studies/grief/index.asp.38 VA, VHA, VISN 19 MIRECC, Neurobiology of Suicide Risk in Traumatic Brain Injury and Substance Abuse, http://www.mirecc.va.gov/visn19 /studies/tbi_sud/docs/tbi_ sud_brochure. pdf.

[39] Suicide prevention is a goal of the Mental Health Quality Enhancement Research Initiative (QUERI) within ORD. See VA Mental Health QUERI Center, Strategic Plan, December 2011, http://www.queri.research.va.gov/about/ strategic_plans/mh.pdf; and VA Mental Health QUERI Center, Fact Sheet, April 2012, http://www.queri. research.va. gov/about/factsheets/mh_factsheet.pdf.

[40] The COE at Canandaigua evaluates implementation of suicide prevention initiatives.

[41] For example, the MIRECC of the VA Rocky Mountain Network is conducting a pilot program to determine whether providing prescription medication in blister packages (rather than bottles) reduces the likelihood of overdose. Veterans Health Administration, Blister Packaging Medication to Increase Treatment Adherence and Clinical Response: Impact on Suicide-Related Morbidity and Mortality, http://www.mirecc.va.gov/projects/ blisterpack/ index.asp.

[42] The War Within, p. 13.

[43] Ibid.

[44] U.S. Government Accountability Office, VA Mental Health: Number of Veterans Receiving Care, Barriers Faced, and Efforts to Increase Access, GAO-12-12, October 14, 2011, pp. 15-17, http://www.gao.gov/products/GAO-12-12.

[45] Ibid. Examples of expanded options include increasing use of telemental health services and call centers (i.e., telephone counseling), integrating mental health services into primary care settings, increasing the number of mental health staff and mental health clinic hours, and adding more Vet Centers.

[46] VA, VHA, Uniform Mental Health Services in VA Medical Centers and Clinics, VHA Handbook 1160.01, September 11, 2008.

[47] U.S. Congress, Senate Committee on Veterans' Affairs, VA Mental Health Care: Closing the Gaps, 112th Cong., 1st sess., July 14, 2011; U.S. Congress, Senate Committee on Veterans' Affairs, VA Mental Health Care: Addressing Wait Times and Access to Care, 112th Cong., 1st sess., November 30, 2011; Gregg Zoroya and Paul Monies, "Lag in Mental Health Care Found at a Third of VA Hospitals," USA Today, November 9, 2011, http://www.usatoday. com/news/military/story/2011-11-09/veterans-mental-health-care/51143216/1; and VHA Mental Health Program Evaluation.

[48] VHA Strategic Plan, Elements 4.1, 4.2, and 4.3.

[49] VHA Strategic Plan, Element 9.1, 9.2, 9.3, and 9.4.

[50] The War Within. Outside the VHA, the term "gatekeeper" (rather than "guide") is generally used.

[51] The War Within.

[52] VHA Strategic Plan, Element 6.2.

[53] VHA Mental Health Program Evaluation, p. 153.

[54] VHA Mental Health Program Evaluation. For example, among veterans for whom maintenance medication is recommended, less than one-third received the recommended continuous treatment (p. 160). Similarly, among veterans receiving psychotherapy, "most did not include elements of an evidence-based modality" (p. 154).

[55] VHA Mental Health Program Evaluation. Less than two-thirds of veterans in a new treatment episode "have a documented assessment of their housing and employment needs" (p. 161). Among veterans with major depressive disorder who were receiving psychotherapy, less than a quarter (23%) "had documentation of an assessment of response to psychotherapy" (p. 155).

[56] Mechanism of injury for suicides among the general U.S. population in CY2007 identified from Centers for Disease Control and Prevention, National Center for Health Statistics. Compressed Mortality File 1999-2007. CDC WONDER On-line Database, compiled from Compressed Mortality File 1999-2007 Series 20 No. 2M, 2010, http://wonder.cdc.gov/cmf-icd10.html.

[57] J. John Mann et al., "Suicide Prevention Strategies: A Systematic Review," Journal of the American Medical Association, vol. 294, no. 16 (October 26, 2005), pp. 2064-2074.

[58] VHA Strategic Plan, Elements 10.4 and 10.6; and VA, Blister Packaging Medication to Increase Treatment Adherence and Clinical Response: Impact on Suicide-Related Morbidity and Mortality, http://www.mirecc.va.gov/ projects/blisterpack/index.asp.

[59] J. John Mann et al., "Suicide Prevention Strategies: A Systematic Review," Journal of the American Medical Association, vol. 294, no. 16 (October 26, 2005), pp. 2064-2074.

[60] VHA Strategic Plan, Element 6.10.

[61] Substance Abuse and Mental Health Services Administration, National Suicide Prevention Lifeline, http://www.suicidepreventionlifeline.org/.

[62] U.S. Congress, House Committee on Veterans' Affairs, Subcommittee on Health, Understanding and Preventing Veteran Suicide, 112th Cong., 1st sess., December 2, 2011, testimony of Jan E. Kemp, RN, Ph.D., National Mental Health Director for Suicide Prevention, Veterans Heath Administration, U.S. Department of Veterans Affairs.

[63] J. John Mann et al., "Suicide Prevention Strategies: A Systematic Review," Journal of the American Medical Association, vol. 294, no. 16 (October 26, 2005), pp. 2064-2074.

[64] National Strategy for Suicide Prevention, p. 63.

[65] J. John Mann et al., "Suicide Prevention Strategies: A Systematic Review," Journal of the American Medical Association, vol. 294, no. 16 (October 26, 2005), pp. 2064-2074.

[66] VHA Strategic Plan, Elements 11.1 and 11.2.

[67] VA, Office of Inspector General, Healthcare Inspection: Evaluation of Suicide Prevention Program Implementation in VHA Facilities, January–June 2009, Report No. 09-00326-223, Washington, DC, September 22, 2009, http://www.va.gov/oig/54/reports/VAOIG-09-00326-223.pdf; and VA, Office of Inspector General, Combined Assessment Program Summary Report: Re-Evaluation of Suicide Safety Plan Practices in Veterans Health Administration Facilities, Report No. 11-01380-128, Washington, DC, March 22, 2011.

[68] Department of Defense Task Force on the Prevention of Suicide by Members of the Armed Forces, The Challenge and the Promise: Strengthening the Force, Preventing Suicide, and Saving Lives, August 2010, pp. 55, 89, http://www.health.mil/dhb/subcommittees-tfpsmaf.cfm; hereinafter referred to as The Challenge and the Promise.

[69] CNAS is a 501(c)3 tax-exempt nonprofit organization located in Washington; it describes itself as independent and non-partisan. See http://www.cnas.org/about.

[70] Margaret Harrell and Nancy Berglass, Losing the Battle: The Challenge of Military Suicide, Center for a New American Security, Washington, DC, October 2011, p. 9; hereinafter referred to as Losing the Battle.

[71] Ibid.

[72] Ibid.

[73] The enrollment file includes veterans receiving benefits from the Veterans Benefits Administration, even if the veterans are not receiving care from VHA.

[74] Han K. Kang and Tim A. Bullman, "Letter: Risk of Suicide Among US Veterans After Returning From the Iraq or Afghanistan War Zones," Journal of the American Medical Association, vol. 300, no. 6 (2008), pp. 652-653. The study was limited to veterans who served in Operations Enduring Freedom and/or Iraqi Freedom and who were separated alive from active duty between October 2001 and December 2005.

[75] See for example Stefan Timmermans, "Suicide determination and the professional authority of medical examiners.," American Sociological Review, vol. 70, no. 2 (2005), pp. 311-333; Hugh P. Whitt, "Where did the bodies go? The social construction of suicide data, New York City, 1976-1992," Sociological Inquiry, vol. 76, no. 2 (2006), pp. 166- 187; M.J. Breiding and B. Wiersema, "Variability of undetermined manner of death classification in the U.S.," Injury Prevention, vol. 12(Suppl II) (2006), pp. ii49-ii54.

[76] Losing the Battle, p. 9.

[77] Ibid.

[78] Charting the Future, p. 40.

[79] U.S. Congress, Senate Committee on Veterans' Affairs, VA Mental Health Care: Closing the Gaps, 112th Cong., 1st sess., July 14, 2011; U.S. Congress, Senate Committee on Veterans' Affairs, VA Mental Health Care: Addressing Wait Times and Access to Care, 112th Cong., 1st sess., November 30, 2011; U.S. Congress, House Committee on Veterans' Affairs, Subcommittee on Health, Understanding and Preventing Veteran Suicide, 112th Cong., 1st sess., December 2, 2011.

[80] Losing the Battle, p. 9; and Charting the Future, p. 40.

[81] Charting the Future, p. 40.

[82] U.S. Congress, Senate Committee on Veterans' Affairs, VA Mental Health Care: Addressing Wait Times and Access to Care, 112th Cong., 1st sess., November 30, 2011; U.S. Congress, House Committee on Veterans' Affairs, Subcommittee on Health, Understanding and Preventing Veteran Suicide, 112th Cong., 1st sess., December 2, 2011.

[83] U.S. Congress, Senate Committee on Veterans' Affairs, VA Mental Health Care: Closing the Gaps, 112th Cong., 1st sess., July 14, 2011. Senator Murray mentioned stigma in her opening statement, and it was discussed at several points.

[84] U.S. Congressional Budget Office, Cost Estimate for H.R. 327 Joshua Omvig Veterans Suicide Prevention Act, March 19, 2007; and U.S. Congressional Budget Office, Cost Estimate for S.4797 Joshua Omvig Veterans Suicide Prevention Act, July 10, 2007.

[85] U.S. Government Accountability Office, Recovering Servicemembers: DOD and VA Have Jointly Developed the Majority of Required Policies but Challenges Remain, GAO-09-728, July 2009, p. 25.

INDEX

D

E

F

G

H

I

J

L

M

N

O

P